Asperger's Syndrome Guide for Teens and Young Adults

Thriving (not Just Surviving)

Plus the following bonus guides:

How to Get Into the College of Your Choice

7 Tips for Success in College with Asperger's Syndrome

Survey to Measure the Bullying Problem in Your School

A Guide to the Individualized Education Program

Craig Kendall

Sign up for Craig's free
Asperger's Syndrome Newsletter at

www.AspergersSociety.org

First published in 2009
by Visions Research
PO Box 1257
Solana Beach, CA 92075

Copyright 2009 by Visions Research

www.VisionsResearch.com

Printed in the United States of America
ISBN 978-0-9841103-1-5

Disclaimer: This information and advice published or made available in this report or web site is not intended to replace the services of a physician, nor does it constitute a doctor-patient relationship. It should not be construed as medical advice or instruction. Information on this web site and in this report is provided for informational purposes only and is not a substitute for professional medical advice. You should not use the information on this web site and in this report for diagnosing or treating a medical or health condition. You should consult a physician in all matters relating to your health, and particularly in respect to any symptoms that may require diagnosis or medical attention. Any action on your part in response to the information provided here is at the reader's discretion. Readers should consult their own physicians concerning the information on this web site or in this report. The publisher makes no representations or warranties with respect to any information offered or provided regarding treatment, action, or application of medication, diagnosis or treatment. The author and Visions Research, LP and Visions Research, Inc. are not liable for any direct or indirect claim, loss or damage resulting from use of this report or web site and/or any web site(s) linked to/from it. The publisher is not responsible for errors or omissions. Reference herein to any specific commercial product, process, or service by trade name, trademark, manufacturer or otherwise does not necessarily constitute or imply its endorsement, recommendation, or favoring by the publisher.

Dedicated to every family and every teenager and young adult – that you find happiness and rewarding, loving relationships

Table of Contents

Bonus Reports

Aspergers is not a curse - it is just a difference, and a difference that can be worked around.

Dear Craig,

It is only now that I realize my daughter who did medicine and is now in general practice has this syndrome, and of course had it as a child. Not much at all was known about Aspergers then, she is now 44 years of age!

I can see from all my reading and knowing my own daughter that she has this syndrome, has no friends, was much more difficult than her sister as a child, has routines, loves animals, works in a cat home on a Sunday morning. She was a very bright, excellent student, had about 2 friends, also very studious, but no longer has contact or very little. I also know now that her father had this syndrome.

This is a poem a boy in her class wrote in her final year at school (they were 17years).

"Litwinner" by B E C

No-one knows where her thoughts lie,
The Quiet Achiever - beautiful, shy.
Courageously toiling, she strives for her goal,
Tenacious Commitment - body and soul.
The work is hard and often long
Her silent labor - steady, strong.
Hers a world of strong devotion,
Modest Brilliance - inspired notions.
The effort she makes is by gentle determination,
Thrashing through her work
Without Procrastination.
Now the time has come when all
rewards are due
to (name withheld) - talented, true.

Section One – Introduction

Hello and welcome. Since you found this guide, you probably have a child or grandchild on the autistic spectrum. Specifically, a teenager with autism. You are probably a bit confused and wondering what to do next, now that your child has hit such a challenging but exciting time in their lives.

All of a sudden, they are not the little kid who needed you all the time. The child who needed you to tie their shoes and cut their grilled cheese sandwich into pieces is replaced by a person with a mind of their own who has their own likes and dislikes, who is exploring the world and finding out how they feel about a variety of different things. This new time might come with extra behavior challenges as they try to push boundaries and limits that they never tried to push before, or it might be a challenge because you feel like you never quite know what is going on in their life.

In this guide, I will describe the issues that you may face, and give you strategies to help you with these issues.

Teenage years can be difficult

The teenage years can be especially difficult for kids with Asperger's syndrome. Of course, every teen is an individual. Some will navigate the rough waters of the teen years better than others. But for some, these years can be extremely difficult. For others, their indifference to what others say and think can shield them from peer pressure and allow them to focus on what they love best ultimately becoming accomplished historians, musicians, mathematicians, or computer professionals.

Poor Social Skills Can Lead to Isolation

A danger during these adolescent years is that your teen becomes increasingly isolated due to their poor social skills. AS teens want friends, they want to date and explore relationships just like any other kid. But middle and high school can be a cruel place for AS teens who may face bullying, rejection and loneliness.

At the same time, school becomes more difficult as teens prepare for college entrance tests. Making the transition from a child to a young adult with all the challenging issues involved – sexuality, relationships, independence from parents – is an especially difficult road to travel for the AS teen.

An issue that is common for AS teens is social isolation. The most common symptom of Asperger's syndrome is poor social skills. And navigating the ever changing relationships of the teenage years is challenging even for those not having AS. Your child may feel like an outcast. He or she may interrupt others, drone on about a subject that they alone find interesting, never make eye contact, or violate others' personal space. Or he may seem nerdy or selfish and aloof because he isn't able to share his thoughts or clearly communicate his ideas or feels with others. As your AS child becomes more isolated and alone, they may act out, mimic negative behavior or turn hostile.

> A danger during these adolescent years is that your teen becomes increasingly isolated due to their poor social skills.

Social Demands on Girls

Many AS teens' speech and actions seem adult-like which will gain few friends in middle school. Or the social demands of teenage girls may simply overwhelm your daughter – the phone calls, the endless chit chat about subjects of little interest – or the constantly changing emotions of the other girls may simply be too much to handle for her.

Not only will many Aspergers teens' actions and behavior alienate them from their peer group, but their blindness to fashion trends may visually isolate them as well. AS teens may neglect hygiene or have uncombed hair – never mind following fashion rules!

Poor motor skills often isolate boys

Boys, in particular, may find it difficult to transition to middle or high school if they have poor motor skills. Playing sports is often an entry key to gaining acceptance and friendship during the teenage years.

Because many AS teens do not fit in, they are not included in the street talk where knowledge and rules of sexuality are often gained. Therefore, they are often very naïve about sexuality. For girls, especially, this can lead to harassment and even date rape.

Loneliness, isolation, depression and an enormous desire to fit in can lead AS teens to associate with the wrong crowd. They may fall into problems with drugs, alcohol or sex. They may become prey for abusive teens who, due to their naivety, get them to buy or carry drugs or alcohol for the group.

While your AS child may have excelled academically in lower grades, middle and high school may pose significant problems. Having to constantly change classrooms, face noisy hallways, have many different teachers – each with his or her own style – can be overwhelming to your child. And with so many teachers, it will be increasingly difficult for a parent to explain to all these teachers the accommodations that your child will need.

Many young people with Aspergers have difficulty staying organized. A long term paper or project may overwhelm them because they do not now how to break down a large project into manageable pieces. And balancing many homework assignments from different teachers can be daunting. One of the greatest hurdles I have had with my son, who has Asperger's syndrome, is just making sure he knows what homework assignments he has. I have had to check his grades, online, and have often found zeros because of missing homework assignments – which he swears were never assigned! Yet all his classmates handed them in.

> Aspergers teenagers often struggle with depression or anxiety as they start to realize how different they are from their peers, and try to make friends or start dating.

Depression and Anxiety

Aspergers teenagers often struggle with depression or anxiety as they start to realize how different they are from their peers, and try to make friends or start dating. Yes, these are challenges common to all teenagers, but to the teenager on the autistic spectrum, it is even more difficult because they have problems understanding social situations, problems regulating emotions, sensory issues, and many other things that get in the way of them being normal teenagers.

Hormonal changes combined with the new stresses of the teenage years can emotionally overwhelm your child. Emotional outbursts can occur. Boys, in particular, may get abusive and physically assault a sibling, teacher or other student. They may melt down after a day of bullying, pressure, harassment, and rejection. As teens have access to cars, drugs and alcohol, real problems can occur resulting in incarceration or involvement with the penal system.

There is hope

But have hope, with proper support, therapy and parents acting as strong advocates, your child can not only survive but thrive. After all, many of us have had difficult teenage years – and pulled through quite nicely. In this book, I will provide solutions, tips and tricks to anticipate and prevent problems before they occur and help you solve those that come out of nowhere.

1. School: Navigating a Changing Environment

School, always a tough issue, right? You fought for your child all the way through elementary school. You got him early intervention when he was little, in the U.S. you fought for Individualized Education Program (IEPs) in the lower grades, and you watched him grow. Or, maybe you're new to all of this, and just got a diagnosis. In that case, you'll be learning how special education works for the first time, learning how to stand up for your child's rights and get the best placements. In either case, it is important to know what your rights are when you are trying to ensure your child gets a good education in middle and high school, just as much as it was earlier.

All kinds of new issues come up when a child gets to junior high. A lot of those are social issues. The social scene gets infinitely more complicated. There are school dances where there might not have been before. Kids start to talk about dating and going out. The rules of friendship change completely. It can be a difficult time. But on the other hand, kids are becoming more independent and in many cases more ready to do things on their own, and that is exciting, too. Also, kids have several different teachers during the day instead of the same one all day, and this is different, too. The work also becomes more complicated and more challenging.

To start our discussion of the needs of teenagers with Asperger's syndrome in school, we will cover some basics that everyone should know about education and Aspergers. These apply to all grade levels; as much to middle and high school as the lower grades.

Importance of a Structured Learning Environment

The most important thing for the adolescent with AS is a structured learning environment with clear expectations, and an environment that is free of sensory distractions, like shouting, whispering kids, or a ticking clock, or other things that might bother them. They might need extra time on tests, material presented in different ways, or aides to help explain social things to them. The class size should be small and as distraction free as possible. Teachers should be patient and be willing to see things and potential problems from the point of view of the AS child.

Aspergers is not a disorder that directly affects someone intellectually. What I mean by this is that it does usually not affect their academic ability. What it does affect is their ability to succeed in a traditional school environment. So, some kids with AS will get along just fine in school without any accommodations. Others will need accommodations, such as aides, quiet places to take tests, more time on tests, and so on.

Establishing an Educational Plan

If your child is deemed to need special education services, testing will be done to see what kind of services your child needs, if any. In the U.S., the law requires schools to develop an IEP, or Individualized Education Program. This document will be written to address your child's unique needs. The government requires that all children receive a free and appropriate education, which means that if they have special needs, they need to be accommodated by law.

If the school is not able to provide for your child's needs, there is a process by which you may be able to get the school to pay for a special school that can. There are many different therapies and accommodations that the school can provide for your AS child. These are decided in the IEP meeting.

An IEP identifies your child's disability and how it affects their involvement and progress in general education curriculum.

Your child's IEP should cover the following:

- Set measurable academic and functional goals.

- Describe of how those goals will be measured and when periodic reports and/or reassessments will be provided.

- List special education services including supplementary aids that are needed to meet the goals.

- List of individual appropriate accommodations necessary to measure achievement (such as extra time needed to take state-mandated tests), and a projected date when services will begin.

- Specifies what services will be necessary to help the child transition to secondary education.

The following are services your child might be eligible for when he attends school, among others:

- Speech therapy

- Occupational therapy

- Special tutoring

- Social skills group therapy

- Perhaps a self contained classroom if necessary

Functional aides may be necessary:

- A computer to help a kid with bad handwriting type

- A tape recorder so the kid can listen to the lectures later

- An aide to help explain what the teacher is saying

These will all be decided on at this meeting. You will present your child's needs, along with anyone else you choose to bring to the meeting, such as an advocate or therapist/doctor of some kind, and together you and the school district will determine what your child needs to be successful in school. A helpful website to learn more about IEP meetings is www.wrightslaw.com. IEP meetings are usually conducted once a year so adjustments can be made to your child's services as he or she changes, if needed.

What if I have difficulty with the school?

For a variety of reasons, AS teens often have behavior problems in school. I am often asked how to get the school to realize that your child is NOT a bad kid. He has a disability with socializing and can't control certain things about his behavior. You must recognize that schools vary. Some are very supportive of learning challenged children and others act like they do not care about these children.

First of all, are you in the U.S.? If not, you will have to check in your country to see exactly which government agencies support children with learning disabilities and follow their rules.

Has your teen been officially diagnosed with Asperger's syndrome (or some other condition) by a recognized professional? If not, you need to start by getting a formal diagnosis. Otherwise, the battle will be uphill.

Now that you have your diagnosis in hand, tell your school that your teen has officially been diagnosed as having a learning disability. Then they have to establish an Individualized Educational Program (IEP) specifically for your child (they have no choice). Make sure you see the special guide to the IEP at the end of this book.

The IEP is developed in concert with the school during a planned meeting. During the process of meeting with the school, the teachers, guidance counselors, and other school officials, I always suggest that you bring your therapist to the meeting. Your teen's therapist knows your child's issues and can explain to the school what special accommodations your child needs.

> Often times we see that AS children are bullied unmercifully in school. They learn that to survive they have to fight back or cause some other type of commotion.

Often times we see that AS children are bullied unmercifully in school. They learn that to survive they have to fight back or cause some other type of commotion. The school is legally obligated to provide a non-hostile learning environment for all learning disabled children. If your child has officially been diagnosed with Asperger's syndrome, then he officially is autistic. Any school will understand a diagnosis of autism (even if many are somewhat behind in their understanding of Aspergers).

I suggest that if your school is not cooperative and does not understand your teen's issues, then you need more ammunition in your corner. This is why I suggest bringing in your child's therapist (or psychologist, psychiatrist, neurologist or whoever diagnosed and knows your teen). This professional can act as a calm third party and bring order to the Individualized Educational Program (IEP) meeting so that it does not turn into a you-against-them meeting.

I suggest that you read the U. S. Government's guide to IEPs (included at the end of this book). It is also at the following site:

www.ed.gov/parents/needs/speced/iepguide/index.html

It has a lot of very valuable information. <u>No parent should go to their IEP meeting without a copy of this.</u>

The introduction to the U.S. Government document on IEPs states:

> Each public school child who receives special education and related services must have an Individualized Education Program (IEP). Each IEP must be designed for one student and must be a truly *individualized* document. The IEP creates an opportunity for teachers, parents, school administrators, related services personnel, and students (when appropriate) to work together to improve educational results for children with disabilities. The IEP is the cornerstone of a quality education for each child with a disability.
>
> To create an effective IEP, parents, teachers, other school staff--and often the student--must come together to look closely at the student's unique needs. These individuals pool knowledge, experience and commitment to design an educational program that will help the student be involved in, and progress in, the general curriculum. The IEP guides the delivery of special education supports and services for the student with a disability. Without a doubt, writing--and implementing--an effective IEP requires teamwork.

What If Parents Don't Agree With the IEP?

> There are times when parents may not agree with the school's recommendations about their child's education. Under the law, parents have the right to challenge deci-

sions about their child's eligibility, evaluation, placement, and the services that the school provides to the child. If parents disagree with the school's actions-or refusal to take action-in these matters, they have the right to pursue a number of options. They may do the following:

- **_Try to reach an agreement._** Parents can talk with school officials about their concerns and try to reach an agreement. Sometimes the agreement can be temporary. For example, the parents and school can agree to try a plan of instruction or a placement for a certain period of time and see how the student does.

- **_Ask for mediation._** During mediation, the parents and school sit down with someone who is not involved in the disagreement and try to reach an agreement. The school may offer mediation, if it is available as an option for resolving disputes prior to due process.

- **_Ask for due process._** During a due process hearing, the parents and school personnel appear before an impartial hearing officer and present their sides of the story. The hearing officer decides how to solve the problem. (Note: Mediation must be available at least at the time a due process hearing is requested.)

- **_File a complaint with the state education agency._** To file a complaint, generally parents write directly to the SEA and say what part of IDEA they believe the school has violated. The agency must resolve the complaint within 60 calendar days. An extension of that time limit is permitted only if exceptional circumstances exist with respect to the complaint.

Many schools simply do not know how to accommodate teens with AS. They may make excuses or simply say that they do not have the resources to help your child. Do not allow the school to get away with this! The law requires that they find the resources and that these resources are customized for your child. As school budgets get cut, schools are reluctant to provide any additional services. Nevertheless, you have to be your child's best advocate and insist that the school provide whatever accommodation your child needs to succeed.

How can I help my teenager succeed in the social environment of middle and high school?

Like I said before, the social scene in middle and high school can be tricky. Often, the peers of a teenager with ASD (autism spectrum disorder, which includes both Aspergers and autism, as well as other related conditions), will mature (from a social skills perspective) much faster than your child. This often leaves the teenager with ASD behind, and it can be very confusing. They might not be able to keep up. In other words, a kid with Aspergers may do all right socially when social activities and interaction is relatively simple, but once they get into the who's dating whom stage of preteens and teens, they can become lost.

All of a sudden all people care about is who is "cool," and who is dating whom. There is a lot of social innuendo that goes completely over their head. Typical adolescents adopt a kind of "social slang" that they tend to speak in, and kids with Aspergers will not understand this. Your AS child might have had a friend that they could have talked about airplanes and rock collecting with, and hung out with, but then when they hit 12 or 13,

> As a parent, it is important to come up with ways that teens with Aspergers and autism can be more involved in the social fabric of their school. This is a major area in which they will need your help.

all of a sudden things change. This friend now wants to know who your Aspie child thinks is cool, and what the latest clothes fashions are, and your Aspie child will have no idea what they are talking about. As a result, your AS teen often will get left behind in their bewilderment.

As a parent, it is important to come up with ways that teens with Aspergers and autism can be more involved in the social fabric of their school. This is a major area in which they will need your help. It is critical to create opportunities where they can interact with their peers in appropriate ways that both will enjoy; ways that make them feel not quite as different.

➢ Social support groups

One thing that can be done is to form social support groups in the school. In other words, take all the kids who are a little bit different and need a little help finding friends, get them together, and provide activities for them to do together. Pizza nights, board games, outside activities, study groups, skateboarding club, whatever they like. Whatever seems to fit the group works. This can be done for any age group and works just as well for teens as it does for younger kids; perhaps even better with teens, because their social skills will probably be a little more developed and they will be more likely to be able to get something out of the group setting. In this way, the child will have a social group that they can feel comfortable with, and practice their social skills at the same time.

➢ Interest groups

Another way to help build social relationships and social skills is to get the teenager with ASD involved in an interest group. There may be groups in the school or community devoted to reading, or playing musical instruments, or chess, or community service, or history – you name it, there's probably a group for it somewhere. If the AS teenager is with other people who share his or her interests, friendships will be more likely to form, and the child will have a place where he feels like he fits in, and a sense of connection.

➢ Develop Social Connection in the School

Find out what the child's skills and strengths are, and use them. Make sure the child has some kind of social connection in school, even if it is only with other teachers. For example, maybe they want to help with copying documents and doing office work in the office; they can develop relationships with the secretaries and office staff, and have some sense of value. Or give them some kind of job in the classroom or school environment that makes them feel useful. If a kid has an interest in technology, they can help in the technology department. Someone gifted in arts can make designs for school T-shirts, posters, or advertisements. And so on. Find a way for the kid to fit in the community somehow. Find a way to make them feel useful.

As teenagers struggle to find a sense of identity, it is even more important than before to find ways to give them activities that will make them feel a sense of value about themselves. AS teens often have low self esteem. This occurs because of the social isolation and continual feedback that they get at school that they are not liked or an outcast. Finding an activity where your teen can build a sense of accomplishment will build their self-esteem.

How can a teacher best help teenagers with ASD learn?

One thing that needs to be addressed is how teachers can best help our teens with autism to learn. They need to know as much about autism spectrum disorders as they can so they understand how to create the best learning environment for them. Teens with autism can easily be distracted by a variety of things: sensory issues, external stimuli other than the task they are supposed to be concentrating on, and so on. They often need to learn in different ways and have things explained to them more thoroughly to understand something. They often get frustrated very easily if they can't understand something right away. If teachers are aware of these issues, they can start to address them.

Advice for Teachers

Teachers should make sure that their classes and instruction is very clear and concrete. Use lots of examples. Use many different methods of explaining something: visual, written, spoken or demonstrated. Hands-on activities to explain a concept can work very well. Be prepared to explain a concept many times. Know that the AS teen thinks very literally, and you might have to work to understand how the AS teen is understanding something you are saying.

Understand that an AS child has many sensory issues and is easily distracted. Don't expect a kid to understand something you are saying if there are people talking nearby, music playing, bright lights, are anything else that might interfere with the child's ability to focus. Try to remove the child to a calm and quiet environment if needed. If the child has a meltdown or becomes upset, it is probably because they are trying to focus on too many things at once and they are overwhelmed. Again, remove them to a calm and quiet place and giver them a chance to relax and calm down. Then, you can try again.

Know that an AS child might often have trouble with things like motor skills, and handwriting can be difficult. Allow them to use a laptop to take notes.

Eliminate Surprises and Create Routine

Try to always have a schedule of what you are going to do in class. Try not to have many surprises, or if you do, expect that the AS child may have difficulty with them. To the greatest extent possible, inform them ahead of time about any changes in schedule. Make sure the teen has a copy of his schedule so they can refer to it at all times. Go over the schedule with them to make sure they are comfortable with it and know what they are supposed to be doing. Many AS teens have difficulty staying organized. Anticipate that an AS teen will need specific training and help with organizational skills. Show the teen how to arrange their notebook; how to write assignments down on a calendar; provide them with organizational tools and demonstrate how to use them. This will go a long way in helping the AS teen succeed and lower their anxiety and frustration levels.

Teachers of individual classes should have a certain way of conducting a class, and stick with it – consistency is key. In middle and high school, someone should help the AS teen keep track of all of their classes, papers, assignments, and so on, and make sure they are not getting lost in the mix. One other possible accommodation: sometimes the AS teen may be late to class because they can't deal with the busy hallways in between classes, and may hang around waiting for them to disperse before going to their next class. Be understanding of issues like this.

What about Grading?

How should an AS child be graded? Well, this depends entirely on the AS child's abilities. Most AS kids, as I said, do fine academically with some added supports, and should be graded by the same academic standards that all students are graded with. There could be some situations in which this isn't appropriate, but that's really up to the child, teacher, and parent to decide if such a situation arises.

If there is a project in which a child is being graded for some kind of social behavior, like working well in a group, their AS limitations should be taken into account, and they should be graded on the academic work they produce instead of their group work. But again, this depends on the child. In some situations, it might be beneficial for the child to learn how to work with a group; in others, it might sim-

23

ply not be possible, and they should be allowed to be excluded from such an activity. Certainly, group work is not a method of teaching that would work well on a regular basis for adolescents with autism or Aspergers.

There might be some cases in which the AS child is given a reduced amount of homework or modified assignments, but otherwise graded the same; this question is impossible to answer further without knowing the unique strengths and weaknesses of the particular AS child.

2. Dating and Puberty

One major issue that comes up in middle and high school is dating and the onset of puberty. Autistic teens typically have the same urges and desires to have relationships and to sexually explore as other teens; the difference is that they often might not understand some of the rules and unspoken guidelines that apply. This can often get them into trouble.

Some teens have trouble knowing when it is appropriate to do things like masturbation, and they need explicit instruction that those things are to be done only in private. Some teens might need to be told that touching any private areas in public is a no no; talking about sexual subjects in public is typically also inappropriate but your AS teen may not understand the bounds.

Girls and Dating

Teenage girls with autism may need special instruction and guidelines to ensure safe dating. They are at special risk for being taken advantage of because they may not understand when someone is harassing them or even abusing them. They might not understand the difference between good attention and bad attention. Again, explicit instruction needs to be given about this issue. Social stories can be written about it, or else just give concrete examples and break it into small pieces so as to be sure you teen understands the concepts you are trying to present.

Another issue that can cause problems with girls is promiscuity. If your AS daughter has few friends, she may be desperate for attention – unfortunately, she may attract the wrong type of attention. All AS teens, boys and girls, tend to interpret what people say literally. They also have a tendency to believe what people say. Girls, especially, may be very naive when it comes to a boy's attention. A smooth talking boy may start complementing your daughter and giving her the attention that she is craving. In a situation like this, your daughter may be very susceptible to manipulation. She may believe whatever the boy tells her. This may lead to early sexual activity or other inappropriate behavior.

Boys and Dating

Adolescent males with autism need to be told rules about how you approach girls in an appropriate way so as not to seem like they are stalkers. Sometimes, caught up in their own enthusiasm and not understanding social rules, teens with AS have been accused of being "creepy" or "bugging" girls, simply because they did not understand how to approach girls in an appropriate way. Also, girls may use indirect language or hints to indicate that your son is moving too fast or that they have little interest in a relationship. Unfortunately, AS teens often misinterpret or completely miss indirect language and hints. For example, a girl may be constantly "busy" when your son asks her for a date; but he may not understand that this is a polite rejection. Unless a girl states flatly that she does not want to date your son, he may continue to call and hound her – creating an unpleasant situation for all involved.

Specific training can avoid problems

Both young women and men can be easily taken advantage of because of their trusting nature and inability to tell the difference between someone who would be good for them and someone who would be bad for them. Both genders should be given instruction about how to recognize if someone is treating them badly, and about how to recognize if someone is compatible with you: for example, Do you have similar interests? Do you enjoy talking with them or doing things with them? Do they treat you well? Does this person ask you for money? Are you buying them gifts but never receive any in return? Teach your AS teen to recognize "red flags" and signs of inappropriate behavior in others.

Instruction should be given very specifically about how to approach a desired person and what words to use when asking for a date or get-together. Include things like body posture, eye contact, word choice, and so on. Also include what not to do, such as not asking repeatedly if the answer is no – and give tips on how to handle rejection. You might want to role play these scenarios with your autistic teenager.

Physical contact

It is important to teach the difference between good touch and bad touch, and to tell your teen to report anything that makes them uncomfortable. Teach them to lock bathroom stalls, and who it is okay to talk about their sexual feelings with and who it is not. Of course these lessons will change as your teen gets older. Teens need to learn that certain behaviors that were okay at an earlier age, like hugging everyone and anyone, or sitting in people's laps, may be inappropriate and send out the wrong messages as they become older. You may find it uncomfortable to be this direct with your child when discussing sexuality, kissing, dating and other romantic subjects. But it is critical to address these issues with your AS teen.

Some teens need to be taught and reminded to do things like shaving and wearing deodorant. Girls will need help learning how to use pads and tampons and learning why they need to do this and why it is important to keep clean when doing so.

The most important thing to remember about teens and sexuality is to provide an open, respectful environment where your teen feels comfortable asking questions – and to provide as much explicit instruction about the ins and outs of dating and social protocols as you can. With a little planning ahead, you can get through this time, and your teen will build the skills and knowledge to navigate the dating world on their own.

Homeschooling

Some teenagers with autism do better when homeschooled. This eliminates the social pressures, and lets them learn at their own rate. It eliminates bullying issues, and lets you tailor a curriculum to their specific needs and interests. Not all parents have the time, energy and ability to do this, but it is something you might consider if your teen is doing poorly in a local school system. Many times parents form home schooling groups where they teach joint lessons to many kids at once, and where the kids can get some socialization with their peers in a more controlled environment. The sensory stimulation of the environment is greatly reduced and there may be more opportunity for therapies that help autism related issues. Many kids on the autistic spectrum can get along fine in regular schools with extra support, but it is just an idea to consider if things do not seem to be going well in a public school setting.

Final Thoughts on Adolescents and School

There are many issues that can and do come up when teens with autism enter middle and high school. Having to get used to an entirely new environment and a new set of social rules; dealing with bullying and teasing, which will be discussed in a later chapter; dealing with more challenging academics; making and keeping friends; depression and anxiety issues, which will also be discussed later; dealing with a burgeoning sexuality and dating. In every case, providing clear and concrete instruction to your teenager about the ins and outs of each issue, and trying to keep the lines of communication open so that your teen will reach out to you when they need help will get you through most of the issues you will encounter.

Counseling may be necessary in some cases to get you through some rough spots; this is normal. Your teen may seem uncommunicative at times and it might be hard to figure out what is going on in their life. This is also normal. Try to find creative ways to encourage communication; respect their feelings, emotions and fears no matter how strange they may seem. Stay in good contact with your child's school and teachers, and try to get as much information as possible from them. If you try to do all of this as much as possible, then your child will be much more likely to have a positive school experience. Remember, you're the parents, you know your child better than anyone. Trust your instincts.

3. Bullying

Unfortunately, one part of life that many people with Aspergers frequently run into, especially in school, is bullying. It is an unfortunate truth that people who are different are going to get noticed in a not so good way by their peers more often than we would like. Bullying is very prevalent in middle and high schools today. It is estimated that 90% of kids with Aspergers will be bullied.

The teenager with Aspergers is particularly prone to bullying issues, because of their social naivety and their lack of knowledge of social rules and skills. They stand out more because they don't know how to blend in. Subtle social nuances are lost on them. They might not know how to dress to fit in, or may not want to. Their voice may be a bit too high, their tone of voice flat, their volume too loud, their word choice a bit off – the smallest of things can set them apart and make them a target for bullies. This can lead to self esteem issues, depression, school anxiety, lack of focus in class, and it can raise other serious issues.

It is important, therefore, to be aware of the different types of bullying that can happen, how to recognize them, and what to do to stop them. It is important to support the victim of bullying; to tell them that the bullying is not their fault; to show them they do have value and teach them self respect. Teachers should be aware of bullying going on in their classrooms and intervene if needed because teens with

AS often will not know what to do to stop the bullying and will be afraid or not know how to ask for help.

In this chapter, we will talk about the different types of bullying; discuss the experience of bullying for teens with Aspergers; discuss the effects of it; and discuss ways to prevent and stop it. We will also discuss ways to help teens who have been bullied recover from the experience of it.

What is Bullying?

There are many different types of bullying, as we have just said. This is something that has been researched quite a bit, and as a general definition of bullying, the consensus seems to be, according to information found on Wikipedia.com:

> "Bullying is an act of repeated aggressive behavior in order to intentionally hurt another person, physically or mentally. Bullying is characterized by an individual behaving in a certain way to gain power over another person (Besag, 1989). Behaviors may include name calling, verbal or written abuse, exclusion from activities, exclusion from social situations, physical abuse, or coercion (Carey, 2003; Whitted & Dupper, 2005). Bullies may behave this way to be perceived as popular or tough or to get attention. They may bully out of jealousy or be acting out because they themselves are bullied (Crothers & Levinson, 2004).
>
> Ross suggests that social aggression or indirect bullying is characterized by threatening the victim into social isolation. This isolation is achieved through a wide variety of techniques, including spreading gossip, refusing to socialize with the victim, bullying other people who wish to socialize with the victim, and criticizing the victim's manner of dress and other socially-significant markers (including the victim's race, religion, disability, etc).

Ross (1998)[8] outlines other forms of indirect bullying which are more subtle and more likely to be verbal, such as name calling, the silent treatment, arguing others into submission, manipulation, gossip/false gossip, lies, rumors/false rumors, staring, giggling, laughing at the victim, saying certain words that trigger a reaction from a past event, and mocking. Children's charity Act Against Bullying was set up in 2003 to help children who were victims of this type of bullying by researching and publishing coping skills."
(http://en.wikipedia.org/wiki/Bullying)

That gives a general overview of what bullying is and what types it can include. Now let's break it down even further.

1. Verbal bullying

This is one of the most common types of bullying. The bully will call the victim names such as "Fat," "Stupid," "Four eyes," "Weird," "Crazy," and so on – or much worse. The bully will often pick an aspect of the victim that they find different, like perhaps if the child has a stutter, and imitate him whenever he sees the child. Or if he has an unusual name, the bully will make up a variation of it and use that. Or the bully might comment on how the child with AS won't have any friends, nobody will ever want to be with them, and so on.

All of these things are very hurtful to the child with AS, who is just starting to develop a self concept and image of themselves. They start to see themselves as worthless and believe that truly no one will ever want to be friends with them. This is perhaps the easiest kind to recognize.

2. Physical bullying

This is when the bully pushes or shoves the kid with AS as they are walking by in the school hallway, just because they can. Or perhaps they might dunk their head into a toilet in the bathroom, or lure them out to some field behind the school and rough them up, kick them, all kinds of awful things have been known to happen to kids at the hands of other kids in schools.

Often the victim is too afraid of the repercussions of reporting on the bully to tell anyone what is happening, so the cycle continues. It is important to try to keep tabs on your teenager and ask him or her about their day and be alert for any change in behavior or affect that seems a bit different. If they start to seem more depressed and withdrawn, bullying could be the reason.

3. Social and Psychological Bullying

There have been studies done to show the difference between bullying in girls and boys. Girls are more likely to use a form of psychological bullying, whereas boys are more likely to use more explicit forms like pushing or shoving or physical means. Psychological bullying is when a group of kids will try to socially exclude the kid with AS from a group; or girls might pretend to invite the AS girl over to their house to hang out, and when the AS teen gets excited, cruelly inform them that they would never do such a thing. They might make prank calls pretending to be a boy asking them out, and then laugh in their faces and say it was a joke. They will do a variety of things to either make the girl feel that she is being included and then shut her out, or else they will be very blatant about shutting her out and telling her she will never be included. They might get their friends to turn against her, spread rumors about her, and do a variety of destructive measures to ensure the girl with AS (or boy, but it's usually girls) knows she is not wanted.

This is very harmful, because the girl gets a very bad picture of herself. She feels very excluded and not wanted, her self esteem plummets, depression and isolation often follows. Again, it is important for a parent to be aware of the teen with AS's moods, social contacts, and general social standing, if possible, to be aware if these things are happening. Counseling is helpful for the teen with AS experiencing this; enrolling them in any kind of group or activity that will bolster their self esteem while enduring this is important; and of course, talking to the school and teachers to figure out how to stop the bullying is important as well.

4. Social media bullying

With the advent of a wide variety of social media like text messaging, the Internet, instant messaging and so on, bullying has spread from just something that happens to kids in school to something that often happens to them when they are home and online as well. Bullies will often IM (instant message) the teen with AS and say cruel things then; they will email them; they will impersonate other people; they will spread rumors about them. This can make the teen feel helpless to stop them.

Sometimes a bully will make an Internet site with false rumors and unpleasant things about a classmate and spread it throughout the whole school. The same can be done with text messaging. There was a case in the news not long ago about a teenage girl who killed herself because of bullying perpetuated by her classmates online. This is not a common end result and is not meant to scare the reader; but parents should be aware of what their teen is doing online and whom they are talking to, to the extent that they are able.

Teens have a limited worldview and often are not able to brush bullying off like adults might; no one likes bullying but due to the limited life experience of teens – and especially the naivety and social immatureness of most AS teens – they take things said against them very seriously and have a hard time believing anything different. Someone saying bad things about them, whether in school or online, is a big deal and can be very distressing. This kind of bullying needs to be stopped. Since online bullying is relatively new, no one has really figured out how to effectively monitor or restrict what is being said on the Internet.

Bullying Prevention Programs

As I said before, bullying can be a very isolating experience. Often a socially inexperienced Aspergers teenager will not know enough about the world and social experiences to even realize that she or he could be or should be treated better, or to recognize that he or she is being bullied, or to know how to ask for help. That is why bullying prevention programs need to be implemented in schools; teachers need to be on the look out for vulnerable students; friendship groups need to be started to support these vulnerable students. It's not just something you can shake off. Kids with AS who are being bullied need to be protected, and given positive influences so that their self esteem is not shattered too badly.

The Effects of Bullying

Bullying can have disastrous effects on both the bully and the victim. Kids who bully others are much more likely to become criminals later on in life and get into trouble with the law when they get older. Teens who are bullied are much more likely to become depressed and even suicidal. They lose self-esteem and their schoolwork often suffers.

One study done in England found that out of 1800 people between the ages of 11 and 18 surveyed, 60% reported having been bullied at one time or another. So bullying is a very prevalent problem.

Coastkid.org reports that 15 to 20 kids every year, that we know of, commit suicide as a direct result of bullying.

So, as you can see, bullying makes kids more likely to engage in a number of harmful behaviors, from suicidal thoughts to alcohol. It also increases absences from school and makes it harder for teens to keep up with their schoolwork. This is especially true for teens with Aspergers who already likely have a lot of anxiety about school and social interactions. If your AS teen is staying home from school often due to illness, you may want to see if bullying is part of the problem.

How Do You Prevent Bullying?

Since bullying is such a big problem for teens with Aspergers, what can we do to protect them and to stop it? There are several programs that innovative school districts have initiated, and much research has been done on the topic of what are the most important components of a successful bullying prevention program. The following are some of the most successful elements.

1. Change the school climate

There are three components to the bullying cycle: the bully, the victim, and the bystander. What a lot of people don't realize is how important the bystander is.

Most witnesses to bullying behavior don't do anything and will not try to intervene to help the victim. They may feel uncomfortable, be afraid that if they try to stop it, they will be picked on next. They may be afraid of seeming uncool. Or they may simply not have the tools needed to know how to stop the bully.

If we are going to change our schools so that our kids with Aspergers are safe, we have to change the climate of the school. It needs to be seen as uncool to bully. Bullies get a lot of silent affirmation from bystanders who do nothing to intervene. It makes them think its okay to bully. Not to mention the bystanders, often their friends, who directly encourage them by egging them on, giving them high fives, and so on.

If bystanders started saying things like "Hey, it's not cool to pick on others," and if bullies didn't get positive reinforcement by seeming "cool" when they picking on others, they would do it less because they would have no motivation to do so.

To this end, it is helpful to hold school wide workshops, where kids role-play the role of the bully, the victim and the bystander, and the appropriate response of each – especially the bystander (those witnessing the behavior). They will learn empathy for others by seeing the plight of the bully, and they will learn how to intervene appropriately when they do see bullying behavior. There are several groups and organizations that come into schools to do workshops and presentations. Try contacting your school's guidance office to see if they could arrange for a workshop such as this; or, develop your own, and ask the school if they could have an assembly to raise awareness of bullying and awareness of why it's important to stop it.

2. Assess the level of bullying at your school

When administrators give surveys to students, staff and teachers, it helps to determine how big of a bullying problem actually exists, therefore helping to shape anti-bullying programs and motivate school personnel to create them. If your school does not survey students, lead the way by getting a sponsor within the school. An empathetic teacher can pass out confidential surveys to students that he or she teaches. A guidance counselor can often generate momentum. A guidance counselor can also enlist the help of the administration and other teachers to implement a survey.

Once facts are gathered, it is then difficult for the school administration to say that bullying is an isolated event or to deny the existence of the problem. With facts in hand you have ammunition. You also have a specific metric. If the survey indicates that 30% of the students have been bullied or witnessed bullying in the past three months, then the school can measure progress with future surveys. If a survey is implemented 6 months later and the number of bullying incidents has not gone down, then the administration can be held accountable for their poor performance. Public school are particularly worried about facts and statistics. School administrators are essentially politicians. They do not want factual data floating around that indicates that they are doing a poor job. If you can prove your case you will have much greater leverage and influence to stop bullying.

As a last resort, report the high percentage to the local press. Local newspapers, in particular, are always interested in data about schools. If you bring a news outlet data that shows that student bullying is a serious problem, it is highly likely that they will report on the problem – which is exactly what the school administration does not want. If the bullying problem can be made public, it is much more likely that it will be taken seriously by the school administration. See the appendix for a sample survey on bullying that you can use in your school.

3. Get parents involved

Parental attitudes are an important part of how their kids act and treat others. Hold meetings with the parents to express to them how important bullying prevention is and ask them to talk about it with their kids. Raising the issue with the Parent Teachers Association (PTA) can also help. Try to find other parents whose children are the subject of unwanted comments, teasing and bullying. There is power in numbers. It will be much more difficult for the school to ignore the problem when they are facing multiple parents, all with the same complaint.

4. Train staff in bullying prevention, and develop clear policies

There needs to be very clear zero tolerance rules in place for bullying, and all teachers and staff need to be trained in how to implement them. Unfortunately, school rules are not always followed or enforced. Many schools have a zero tolerance policy for bullying, but bullying is still rampant. This often happens because teachers do not take an active enough roll in preventing it. They may also be unaware of the problem because they are not actively looking for acts of bullying. And what is bullying? A teacher may see a student bump into another student and then laugh. The teacher may not realize that this is one element in a continuing string of harassing events. Since the teacher only sees this singe event, they may think to themselves that the kids are just "fooling around." The teacher may not realize that the person is being continually tormented by this constant harassment.

Bullying is typically a problem when it is on-going, when the bully taunts and continues to harass another student over a period of time. A teacher seeing one isolated incident may not realize that they are witnessing a well planned campaign of harassment. Programs to teach teachers how to respond to seemingly isolated incidents can go a long way in identifying and preventing bullying.

5. Increase adult supervision in areas where bullying occurs the most

There tends to be more bullying in areas not as closely observed by teachers or other adults. Lunchrooms, locker rooms, busy hallways and so on should all be more closely monitored if possible for bullying behavior. Bullying behavior should be stopped immediately if seen.

6. Incorporate bullying prevention themes into the classroom

Experts suggest setting aside twenty or thirty minutes every week to discuss issues of bullying and peer relations in the classroom. This can help teachers keep an eye on how things are going in the school and address any issues that need addressing. It also reinforces the lesson that bullying will not be tolerated, and that treating your peers with respect is very important. Obviously, this is easier to do in the younger grades when kids are in one class all day, but it can also be done in homerooms of middle and high schools once a week, for a short time.

If a school incorporates these ideas, they will be well on their way of greatly reducing the amount of bullying in their school. It's all about changing attitudes and making school a safe place to learn for its most vulnerable citizens. Teens with Aspergers have enough problems already without being subjected to harassment and abuse by their peers on a regular basis. We need to do something about this problem. We need to give everyone the tools they need to succeed and feel safe. Implementing programs such as the one above is one great way to start.

Traumatized Teens: How To Help Your Teen with Aspergers Cope and Recover from Bullying

Unfortunately, sometimes our best efforts at preventing bullying fail. It's just too prevalent, and it's hard to monitor every inch of a school that often has a thousand or more students. So, what do you do if you know your kid is being bullied? How do you help him or her recover?

The first step

The first thing you should do if you suspect your teen is being bullied, is schedule a meeting with the school and his teachers to discuss the matter. Ask them what they have observed. Ask them if there is anything you can change about his schedule to make it less likely that the bullying will happen. Perhaps he can leave class 5 minutes early or late to avoid the rush that goes on in the hallways and not be as likely to run into the bullies? Perhaps an aide can be assigned part time to help him navigate the social waters? Perhaps a bullying prevention program can be designed for the school? Ask the teachers to be more vigilant about watching out for your teen and to intervene if they see bullying happen. After all, teachers want to help your child. If they are made aware that your child is being bullied and if they understand the deep hurt and depression that is being caused, they are likely to be more diligent in observing and preventing the problem. Elicit as much help as possible and build as large a team as you can to help your child.

Support your teen by making sure he or she knows you are there to support them and that they can always talk with you about what they have been through or other problems they may be having. Support their sense of self-esteem by enrolling them in activities or groups where they will be surrounded by people who will respect them and appreciate their gifts and strengths. One way to do this is by considering their interests and trying to find groups related to it.

Therapy often helps

Consider therapy to help them deal with the self-esteem blow and identity questions they are dealing with. Counseling can be a safe place for them to discuss what is happening to them and talk it out with someone who can understand and help them make sense of it. Someone who can help them see that the bullying isn't their fault, that they did nothing to deserve it. Someone who can help come up with coping techniques for dealing with bullies in the future. There are many benefits of a good counselor for any teen with Aspergers. Learning skills to navigate the social world is important in itself but these skills become essential to help a teen who is experiencing bullying.

As parents we love and appreciate our kids. But how often do we tell them that? Unfortunately, all too often, we focus on "correcting" negatives or perceived bad behavior while spending much less effort and energy focusing on positives and good behavior. Make sure you constantly praise their strengths and good points to counter the messages they are getting from the bullies. Below is a list of positive messages that you should be saying at least daily to your teen.

Complements to Build Your Teen's Self-Esteem

- Good for You
- How did you do that?
- That's really nice
- Keep up the good work.
- That's quite an improvement.
- Thank you very much.
- That's clever.
- Congratulations!
- Now you've got the hang of it.
- Terrific effort!
- Super!
- Beautiful!
- You've got it now.
- Nice Going
- I appreciate what you've done.
- That's coming along nicely.
- That's going to be great.
- I like the way you...
- I'm glad that you're my son.
- You're a good leader.
- It looks like you put a lot of work into this.
- Thanks for your cooperation

Effects of Bullying Can be Long-lasting

Unfortunately, all too often, the effects of bullying are long-lasting. Some people are resilient enough and grounded enough in their own self worth to be able to withstand bullying behavior without being emotionally scarred; but many carry the memories and experience of being bullied into adulthood. It can shape their image of themselves and their expectations of how others will treat them for years to come.

Even after the bullying has stopped, many teens remain traumatized by it. They become afraid of people, unsure of themselves, or sure that every person they meet is secretly making fun of them behind their backs. They may develop extreme school avoidance or anxiety about school. They may have a hard time getting close to others in the future because they are so afraid of being hurt. Again, people with AS have a hard enough time being confident socially without being bullied. But when bullying happens, it's a bit of a double whammy and affects their idea of how they are able to function socially.

Surround your child with positive experiences

It may take as much as a few years or even longer after the teen is removed from the bullying environment for them to get their self esteem and sense of self back. Your child needs to be surrounded by positive experiences and needs positive social interactions for them to start healing. When they start to learn that people might actually like them for who they are; when they start to see that they don't need to change themselves for people to like them; when they start to see that people will approach them and say hi to them and be friends with them just because of who they are — that is when they can start to heal and become more confident about themselves and their social abilities.

A key to countering the effects of bullying while building self esteem is to put your teen into environments where they will be likely to succeed. For instance, if they have an interest in writing, find a writing summer camp that has others interested in writing. Teens interested in more intellectual pursuits often tend to be kinder and more mature than their peers – not always but often. Look at summer camps run by a college where the campers take classes – these are often run for high school students wanting to get a taste of what college will be like. Again, the maturity level will be higher, and your teen has a much better chance of making friends and finding kinder, like minded people that can start to let them heal from the abuse in their past. The transformation can be incredible to watch. Once they find their wings, so to speak, they realize what they are able to do. It's just a matter of finding the right kind of place with the right kind of people.

Summer camps that have a selective application process are even better as the participants have already been screened. Many colleges run programs like this. Teens with Aspergers are often interested in subjects like science, psychology, or other academic pursuits, so summer camps dedicated to these areas of interest, with peers who actually want to be there and want to be learning these things as well, can be ideal for the teen with Aspergers.

Sometimes, it just takes getting out of the high school environment for the teen who has been bullied to be able to flourish. It takes perhaps going to a college with a much more tolerant student body, or getting a job and experiencing professional success, for a person to finally get beyond the bullying in their past. It can be a long and arduous process, but it can be done.

BULLYING FROM THE PERSPECTIVE OF A YOUNG ADULT WITH ASPERGERS

When researching for this chapter, I came across this piece written by a young woman with Aspergers that I would like to share with you, as a message of hope for all your teens who are experiencing bullying. This woman had experienced a lot of bullying in her past and had been very adversely affected by it. In her mid-20s, however, she was finally able to get to a place where she was mostly at peace with it. She realized she was a stronger person for having endured it, and that she had a much stronger sense of self in the end for having had to work so hard to figure out who she was. She took a lot of pride in finally being able to say that she recognized her self-worth, was proud to be who she was, and she wasn't going to let anyone ever make her feel ashamed for who she was again.

For all the socially inept teens with Aspergers who have lost their way and their sense of self because of the bullying done to them, this is a message of hope to them. This might be something you want to share with your teen if they are experiencing this; more stories of hope and healing can most likely be found online as well. Not all stories end well, but some do.

"The Ice Cream Incident," (the writer asked to remain anonymous)

***

On a bright, sunny and beautiful afternoon, I was making my way up a busy road, headed for an ice cream place in Newport. I had my Walkman on and was enjoying the music, the sunshine, and the high that comes from actually knowing where I was going. It was a new town that I had just moved to, and I was used to getting lost. I had a smile on my face and was almost there, when someone shouted "Hey!" and I looked up, automatically. A derogatory comment followed, a man in a car with the windows down zipping by. Let's just say it started with weird and ended with a word that rhymes with witch.

My first reaction, I am happy to report, was of pity for the man. Here I was, walking to an ice cream place, enjoying a sunny day, enjoying life, and his life was obviously so miserable that he had to get joy out of yelling insults at strangers. I mean, honestly, how happy can a man who needs to entertain himself by yelling at strangers from moving cars be? Such a person obviously has major insecurities, major self esteem issues, major satisfaction with life issues. It's pitiful, really, it's a shame. It's degrading – to him, not me. It's a reflection on the kind of person he is and the life that he leads – not on me.

It was at that moment that I realized my life was rich, and that his was not. It was that point I realized, I had found ways to make myself happy in life, despite my many challenges. I didn't need much. I just needed a sunny day and an Ice cream place. He, on the other hand, our nameless road rage guy, needed to put down others to get his jollies. Again, what a miserable existence. I thought I was poor, yet I found I was rich.

I also can't pretend the comment didn't hurt at all. That would be foolish to do. It still did, a little, but it was maybe 70% feeling sorry for him and even amused that someone would find it necessary to do such a thing – is my joy threatening to him? Does the prospect of happiness in the world, the idea of happiness overtly expressed, scare him? I have come too far in my life, I have worked way too hard on accepting myself, on finding ways to access the world, to accommodate my difficulties and find ways to participate, and even participate happily, in the world to let someone rain on my parade now.

And that is the other thing that I realized as I thought about this incident (but not, of course, until after I had made my way to the ice cream place and enjoyed some espresso ice cream and some more sunshine). Pride in realizing how far I have come, and pride in realizing that I am indeed strong in the broken places. It is not so much of a stretch to remember what I used to be like. I don't like to do it, but I can. I can remember the me who used to be terrified of others, terrified of everyone I met,

47

sure that every one of them was laughing behind my back, telling stories about me to their friends, about to turn on me in any second. I lost my trust in people for a good long time after my junior high and early high school experiences. I was traumatized and afraid. Years of bullying had left its mark. I had no self-esteem, I was afraid to breathe wrong, walk wrong, talk wrong, and so on. I was paranoid about what people thought about me.

But, you know what I think saved me is my basic sense of integrity to myself. I always knew there was no sense in changing yourself to please others. The reasons are obvious. So I didn't. I withdrew from people, became terribly isolated, lonely and depressed, but I never stopped being true to who I was. I never stopped expressing my thoughts, wearing what I wanted to wear, listening to what I wanted to listen to, thinking what I wanted to think. And years later, when I finally got around a group of people who could accept me for who I was, accept every quirk, accept every difference, they healed the broken spots. They restored my ability to trust in people again. They restored my sense of self-esteem, my sense of connection to others. And they gave me permission to be myself and be proud of it. I learned not to be ashamed of myself.

Because of the bullying, for several years, I lost my ability to be a part of the world around me, in a sense. I wasn't an exceedingly social person before this happened, a lot which could be attributed to my Aspergers diagnosis, but the peer abuse took away my ability to see myself as a person in relation to others.

So what happened, and how did I find my way back? It was such a long process, that I couldn't have told you it was happening when it was. My first year or two of college, I was scared and skittish and had awful flashbacks of mistreatment by peers in previous times whenever I'd get near, well, anyone my age. Which, you know, is kind of a hard thing to deal with in a college environment when you're surrounded by other college students. I had massive self-esteem issues and regularly entertained sobbing fits when I compared myself to others.

By my junior year or so, I realized something. No one had made fun of me in two years. No one had given any

48

indication of being uncomfortable around me. Hell, people had even given me compliments. They said my joy was contagious. They said I was smart, I was a good person to be around. I was compassionate, and cared about others. I realized I could be as quirky as I wanted, I could wander around singing at the top of my lungs, I could do whatever, be whatever, and no one would give me a second glance. No one ever commented on how weird or strange I was. I stopped looking behind my back; I stopped worrying about what people thought; I gained my sense of my self back. I became far more confident about engaging in conversations, about participating in anything social. I began to think when someone talked to me, it was because they actually WANTED to talk to me, not because they were dared to talk to me by their friends. I realized finally that I was an okay person. I was a good person. Sure, I had my strengths and weaknesses like any other person. I was far from perfect. But I was okay. I was a worthy person. Eight years later, I know that my value is not measured by someone else's actions. I still have my problems, but I am more okay with myself than I thought I ever could be.

Anonymous

***

Our kids have many issues. Sensory issues, lack of social skills, need for routine, and trouble understanding what is expected of them. It is disheartening, to say the least, that they have to so often suffer so much abuse from simply being who they are. Their lack of knowledge of social cues and social understanding makes them all too vulnerable to being singled out for bullying. We should take heart in the above story knowing, however, that the damage is not permanent – of course, no one wants their child to suffer like that, and for so long. So we can take this as a message, then, that we need to do what we can to reduce bullying in schools, to recognize when it's happening, and to take steps to eliminate it. We can take steps to support our kids when they are going through it, and steps to educate the community and world around us on what bullying is and what the dangers are. Knowledge is a good thing. Armed with a little knowledge, we can help our Aspergers kids succeed in the world.

4. The Dangerous New Menace – Cyberbullying

Bullying. It's a tough topic. Most have experienced it in some way, or know someone who has. The disastrous effects bullying can have on teenagers and, in fact, anyone are well documented. When parents think of bullying, they typically think of the most traditional forms of bullying like verbal insults, physical bullying such as pushing someone into a locker, kicking them, or attacking them; and social forms of bullying such as exclusion from social circles, spreading rumors about them and so on. By now you should be aware, too, that bullying can lower self esteem in the victim, cause depression, anxiety and even sometimes lead to suicide. Bullies are more likely to have trouble with the law later on. It's a difficult problem, and one that no one has come up with a perfect solution to yet; no matter what, it seems to be very prevalent in all areas where people, especially young people, gather.

But did you know that there is another form of bullying that takes place without any people being present? A form of bullying where you don't even have to be in the same state as the bully to be a victim? A kind of bullying that is perhaps even more insidious than the traditional forms, because it can occur in the victim's own house, in their bedroom, even as they are about to go to sleep? Even as they are on vacation in another city? It's called cyberbullying. Cyberbullying is a relatively new phenomenon that occurred with the rise of all the technology we now have. Cyberbullying can and is done using emails, instant messagers, chat rooms and even cell phones.

What is cyberbullying?

Cyberbullying usually consists of harassing messages that one teenager sends to another, using any of these mediums. A 13 year old girl may sign on after a day of school to find messages such as "You're fat," "Everyone thinks you're awful," "You don't deserve to be alive," or other cruel insults. She may sign into her email to find that a classmate has circulated vicious rumors about her. "Abby slept with John." "Abby is a slut." "No one likes Abby." "Abby is a lesbian." And so on. Or she might receive these things by text message on her cell phone. As technology has increased, so has the ability of all of us to be able to contact those that we know, wherever they are, at any time. Technology makes us tethered to the world around us 24/7. Sometimes, that is not always a good thing.

According to StopCyberBullying.org, "Cyberbullying" is when a child, preteen or teen is tormented, threatened, harassed, humiliated, embarrassed or otherwise targeted by another child, preteen or teen using the Internet, interactive and digital technologies or mobile phones. It has to have a minor on both sides, or at least have been instigated by a minor against another minor. Once adults become involved, it is plain and simple cyber-harassment or cyberstalking. It isn't when adults are trying to lure children into offline meetings, that is called sexual exploitation or luring by a sexual predator. But sometimes when a minor starts a cyberbullying campaign it involves sexual predators who are intrigued by the sexual harassment or even ads posted by the cyberbullying offering up the victim for sex."

Prevalence and Significance of Cyberbullying

According to a recent survey in 2007 ...

- 17% of a 2,000 student middle school reported being cyberbullied

- 43% (almost half of all students) reported the following things having happened to them recently:

    o Received an e-mail that made them upset (not spam)

    o Received an instant message (IM) that made them upset

    o Had something posted on MySpace that made them upset

    o Been made fun of in chat room

    o Had something posted on a Web site that they didn't want others to see

    o Been afraid to go on the computer

A study done by the *National Institute of Health* found that one in ten kids in grades 6 through 10 have either bullied classmates or been bullied by them, online or through cell phones. A study published in the *Journal of Adolescent Medicine* shows:

- 21% reported being a victim of physical bullying

- 53% of verbal bullying

- 51% social bullying, i.e. social exclusion

- 14% cyberbullying

This shows that although cyberbullying at this time might be a less common form of bullying than the other forms, it is gaining speed and becoming a major issue for kids.

Why is Cyberbullying often worse than regular bullying?

1. Cyberbullying has the potential to go viral.

You can send hundreds of text messages spreading rumors about a person out to your classmates in about two minutes. You can email a hundred girls to tell them someone is gay in thirty seconds. Compared to writing something on a bathroom wall, this is huge. The potential audience that gets these messages is huge. The effects can be disastrous. There is no way to protect yourself.

2. Lack of face to face aspect

It is much easier to say something hateful about someone else when you're not looking at them. The perceived anonymity of the Internet makes some bullies feel much more powerful and much less afraid to say whatever they want about whoever, at any time. There is less of a feeling of accountability. There is little risk for feelings of guilt, when you're staring at a computer screen.

3. Less Supervision

Most kids are completely unsupervised when it comes to computer use. There is no chance of a teacher or monitor walking into the locker room, bathroom or lunchroom to see and stop the bullying while it is in progress.

There is no hope for repercussions to the bully because it is all done underground. Adults are usually not aware that cyberbullying is happening at all. There is no one to stop it.

4. It happens in isolation

The victims are bullied in the privacy of their own rooms. They may feel that there is no one to turn to. They may decide to take rash actions without anyone ever knowing anything is wrong. There is little possibility for intervention if no adults know that it is happening.

Steps to protect your children

Teens who are bullied online or by text message are subject to just as much depression, anxiety and other issues as those bullied in the traditional way. There have been cases of kids who were cyberbullied killing themselves. It is an issue that needs to be taken seriously.

The following are two important steps that parents should take to protect their children.

1. Monitoring your kid's emails, instant messages and text messages is a good first step, so that you know what is happening in your teen's life.

2. Talking to them about cyberbullying so that they know what it is and how to deal with it when it happens is another good idea.

Forms of Cyberbullying

You may be thinking to yourself "Where do I start?" Many parents are very unfamiliar with cyberbullying. While many parents can name a few of the possible forms of cyberbullying, most parents are totally unaware of all the possible electronic avenues a cyberbully can use. After all, how can you monitor your kid's activities if you don't know they even exist? Parents must become educated and aware of all of the possible avenues that a cyberbully may use to attack your child.

What are the different forms of cyberbullying?

Email consists of messages sent by electronic mail from one person to another.

Instant messaging services are free services your child can sign up for; they put their "buddies" online and when they are both online at the same time, they can send messages to each other in real time.

Chat rooms are windows in which people can talk to each other in real time, similar to instant messaging but with more people. The language used is often vulgar depending on which chat rooms you go to. There are chat rooms for hundreds of different topics and interests, and there are some chat rooms just for people to hang out in with no particular topic. These tend to attract a population that is more potentially dangerous than chat rooms dedicated to particular subjects.

Message boards are websites where you can post a message about various topics; others can come by, view the message, and post something of their own.

Websites are pages on the Internet with static information that everyone can view.

Text messages are words, numbers, or combinations of letters and slang that can be sent from one cell phone to another instantly.

Polling Sites: Some websites allow you to create polls and voting on questions of your own choosing. For example, a student can set up a page that lets people vote for the fattest, ugliest, sluttiest, etc. boy or girl at their school; using the above messages, the web page can be publicized and gain many votes very quickly.

As you can see, there many ways in which teens can use recent technology to bully and pick on each other when they are not face to face.

The National Crime Prevention Council is currently running ads on the radio trying to raise awareness of cyberbullying and how to prevent it. They list the following forms that cyberbullying can take:

Cyberbullies will:

- Pretend they are other people online to trick others
- Spread lies and rumors about victims
- Trick people into revealing personal information
- Send or forward mean text messages
- Post pictures of victims without their consent

When teens were asked why they think others cyberbully, 81 percent said that cyberbullies think it's funny. Other teens believe that youth who cyberbully

- Don't think it's a big deal
- Don't think about the consequences
- Are encouraged by friends
- Think everybody cyberbullies
- Think they won't get caught

It seems there are an awful lot of ways to spread negative information about someone online, and there is a huge lack of awareness about how damaging this can actually be.

Experiences of Kids, Preteens and Adolescents with Cyberbullying

The Cyberbullying Research center has gathered together many stories and testimonials of those who have experienced cyberbullying. A theme of shame, humiliation and pain, as well as a sense of vulnerability, run through most of these kids' stories. (www.cyberbullying.us)

A 12 year old girl from Virginia expresses that, "Being bullied makes me feel really bad, and I often get depressed later at home. I would also plot revenge and privately express my 'hatred' towards the bully, but I doubt I would really do anything about it...I don't usually go to adults to 'tattle' on people, even though I know it's not tattling, it's real."

A 15 year old boy from New Jersey reveals that, "My friend's friend started to make fun of my ethnic background, so I told him to stop disrespecting me. He ignored my plead and started to get even more verbally abusive. I ignored him but he started talking to me saying that I shouldn't f***k with him because he would beat my a** down in front of his friends."

Some talk about how much harder it is to be bullied on the Internet:

"Being bullied over the internet is worse. It's torment and it hurts. They say "sticks and stones may break my bones, but words will never hurt me." That quote is a lie and I don't believe in it. Sticks and stones may cause nasty cuts and scars, but those cuts and scars will heal. Insulting words hurt and sometimes take forever to heal."

And some talk about the power of words to stick around and cause damage:

"I still cry when I think of what she said. After awhile you start believing all of the things people tell you that aren't

58

true. When I look in the mirror I wonder if I'm fat (I'm not) after what my ex-friend said."

"But I know because I have myself been bullied. It lowers my self-esteem. It makes me feel really crappy. It makes me walk around the rest of the day feeling worthless, like no one cares. It makes me very, very depressed."

Cyberbullying, it seems, can often cause depression and trouble with concentrating in school in its victims:

"It makes me feel bad and rather depressed. Like I don't want to be a part of this world any more."

"One of my friends started hassling me on MSN messenger; she was sending me nasty messages and text messages and this carried on at school. I told my parents, my friends, and a teacher. She was spoken to a few times but it still carries on a bit now but not as bad because I have blocked her online. This really affected me at home and at school; I couldn't concentrate on school work and I was always upset and down; now I just ignore it and get on with it, I have plenty more friends and I don't need her anymore. Maybe one day she will give up and grow up."

Many times, it seems, kids will switch roles of bully and victim depending on their moods. One week, a teen will bully someone on online, and the next week they will be bullied themselves.

"Well the only reason I bullied is because the same person I was doing it to, did it to me like a week before. It wasn't the right thing to do but at the time it felt like I was getting revenge."

Tom Woods says this of his cyberbullying experience:

"It continues 24/7, no matter where they are, they will be hurt, the audience can indeed make them feel violated, and the ability for the abuse to be read or watched again and again just amplifies the impact. It's normal bullying times 3."

Effects of Cyberbullying

As the above stories illustrate, cyberbullying can erode self esteem, cause depression and anxiety, take away the one place a teen feels safe (their home); it can cause irritability and trouble concentrating in school; it can even lead to thoughts about suicide. Even though there is no physical contact in cyberbullying, it can have psychological and emotional impacts and damage on youth. Victims often feel hurt, sad, embarrassed, afraid and lonely.

Preventing Cyberbullying

Well, now you know what cyberbullying is, but how do you prevent it? What as parents and school officials can we do? How can we educate our teens so they won't take part in this menace? There are several things you should know.

First of all, the key in preventing cyberbullying is education. Kids, teachers, parents all need to know what cyberbullying is and ways to prevent its spread.

12 tips for teens to prevent and deal with the spread of cyberbullying:

1. Never give out passwords

Never give out your password to anyone; don't give out other people's passwords to your friends.

2. Make it hard to figure out passwords

Make it hard to figure out passwords and secret questions with unique answers so people can't get into your accounts and use them to send fake email from you and so on.

3. Be careful about what you say online

Be very careful about what you say online about others, because what you say can be understood differently than you intend it. Don't say negative things about your peers online. Don't ever say anything that you wouldn't want passed on to a hundred of your closest friends.

4. Don't start a cyberbullying war

Don't incite bullying by insulting others online.

5. Don't keep quiet if you are being cyberbullied

Tell your friends if you are offended by something or if something goes too far.

6. Turn on comment moderation when possible

If a site you are posting on has comment moderation, turn it on, so offensive comments don't get posted.

7. Stand up for yourself.

If someone is bullying you online, tell someone: a parent or teacher to let them know.

8. Don't play into the cyberbully's hand by responding

If someone is taunting you online, try not to respond if you can, as it will often only make things worse and escalate things. If you don't give them the satisfaction of a response, it will often take their motivation away to bully.

9. Report any abuse of services to service providers

If someone is harassing you online, they can be reported and hopefully dealt with by the service provider. Save all evidence of any bullying online.

10. Don't open emails from anyone you don't know.

Don't give out personal information to anyone online; not in blogs, chat rooms, websites, profiles or any other form of online media.

11. Don't send emails when you're angry

Think to yourself how it would feel to get the email you are about to send. If you wouldn't like it, don't send it.

12. Help others who are being cyberbullied

Help others who are being bullied online by not participating in the bullying and showing bullying messages to an adult.

Six Steps Parents Can Take to Prevent Cyberbullying

1. **Keep your family computer in a busy area of the house** so you can observe what your child is doing, and their response to any messages they might get.

2. **Set up your kid's email and instant messaging services** so you know their password and can keep an eye on things.

3. **Discuss cyberbullying with your child.** Make sure they know what it is, how to respond and to talk to you about it if it ever happens to them.

4. **Tell your kids that if they are cyberbullied, you won't take the computer from them.** A lot of kids don't tell their parents about cyberbullying because they are worried about the computer being taken away from them if they tell what is happening to them. This is one major thing that prevents kids from getting help when they are bullied.

5. **Go over your kid's instant message list** with them to make sure you, and they, know who everyone on it is.

6. **Be supportive of your child** when he or she reports being cyberbullied. It might not seem like much to you, but it can have lasting effects on your child.

What the School Can Do to Help Prevent Cyberbullying

Schools should take an active role in preventing and setting rules about cyberbullying. Some schools have clauses in their Internet use contracts that students are responsible for and accountable for their behavior online both in school and *off* school grounds. This way they can lose privileges and be punished at school for engaging in bullying behavior off school grounds. Many schools ban the use of cell phones in school so that bullying by text message can not occur.

It is important to have awareness programs; hold lectures and assemblies on what cyberbullying is, why it is bad, and how to prevent it; spreading the message to the kids who engage in it will help educate them and hopefully spur them to stop or reduce their cyberbullying. Some kids do not realize what they are doing when they cyberbully; some don't realize the effect they are having on others. Some do it for a feeling of power; some do it for revenge; some do it just because they are angry or because it was done to them. The cycle needs to stop, and education is the best way to stop it.

The website HotChalk.com summarizes this issue nicely by giving ten very important tips on how to prevent cyberbullying:

1. Tell students to never pass along harmful or cruel messages or images.

2. Train students to delete suspicious email messages without opening them.

3. Ask students to step up to friends who are cyberbullying and tell them to stop.

4. Teach students how to use technology to block communication with cyberbullies.

5. Speak to students about the importance of telling a parent or adult about any cyberbullying they're witness to.

6. At home, supervise your child's time online. Putting the computer in a common area, such as the kitchen, is a good idea.

7. Addressing cyberbullying school-wide is key – help institute a formal policy for dealing with any cyberbullying instances. Be sure students fully understand the consequences. For some guidelines on crafting a program, visit HotChalk.com and see Preventing Cyberbullying: A Conversation with Mike Donlin.

8. Create a community outreach program to educate those beyond the school walls to the dangers of cyberbullying. Have students work with the Chamber of Commerce or other civic group to create an awareness campaign.

9. Teach students the basics of smart and savvy Web behavior, such as never revealing passwords or real last names.

10. Pay attention. If you notice a student is withdrawn, depressed or reluctant to attend school or social events, investigate.

With enough vigilance and understanding about this topic, hopefully we can stop the spread of cyberbullying.

Cyberbullying in the news

One indicator of how big an issue cyberbullying has become is its prevalence in the news lately. Below are just some snippets of recent stories about cyberbullying in the news.

One of the biggest cyberbullying stories in the news lately has to do with a young girl named Megan Williams. Megan was 14 when she killed herself over stress from an online exchange of messages. A boy named Josh had contacted her and they developed a quick friendship; but after a while, Josh started insulting her and saying things like "I don't want to be friends with you anymore; you're a slut; you're fat." Devastated and not able to understand why her friendship had unraveled so fast, Megan took her life.

This story shows the need for transparency in online communications for parents, and also the need to educate kids on how online friendships are different from real life friendships.

In another story, two law students were subject to what is equivalent to a modern day "stoning" online. In a popular law message board, the two had all kinds of vile things said about them. When they do a Google search for their names, these things come up. This is of course damaging to their professional reputation, for anyone who may be looking to hire them, damaging to their self esteem, humiliating and painful to read.

Brittan Heller and Heide Iravani had multitudes of comments posted such as that Heller has herpes and had bribed her way into Yale, helped by a secret lesbian affair with the dean of admissions, or that Iravani was a heroin addict and had sex for the dean in exchange for a passing grade. They are attempting to sue the individual perpetuators for defamation and emotional distress.

According to eschoolnews.com, "a Portage, Ind., high school student was accused of threatening the life of another student over the internet – and in San Francisco, an unidentified student reportedly hacked into a high school web site, posted a student's face over vulgar and mocking images, then added racist captions using the victim's name." But everyone from the federal government to local school districts are trying to fight back.

"The federal government, for instance, recently added information about cyberbullying to the $3.2 million "Stop Bullying Now!" campaign that it launched last year. The Beaverton, Ore., school system is revising its health curriculum, and cyberbullying is among the topics that officials there might include. Cyberbullying also has been added as a topic in many internet safety courses, such as the free lessons from i-SAFE America Inc. "

The Sun reported on teenagers who had been cyberbullied. Georgia Woods' story, a 13 year old who lives in Kentucky, rings particularly poignant given everything we have said so far. Her story is unfortunately far too common:

"I didn't tell my mum at first as I didn't want to worry her. Home is where you're supposed to feel safe, but instead I was upset and scared. I started to wonder if what they were saying was true, and it got to the stage where I had no friends at school. I'd eat my lunch quickly on my own, then run to the toilets and cry. When I was at home on my own I'd switch all the lights off and just scream. I even put my school tie around the toilet door to try to hang myself, but couldn't go through with it. "

The Sun also reports on the case of now 19 year old Julianne Flory, whose parents had to go to the police to stop cyberbullying. She reports,

"By the time I turned 15 they were targeting me on the internet. I'd built a personal website for my friends to access. One day I found the message page littered with insults. There were various comments about my appearance, another posting said I was a lesbian and that they hoped I'd die a slow and painful death. Threats were common. On one occasion the user said they'd like to pull my fingernails out. I was upset and scared. It was bad enough facing them in school, but now they could get me in my own home. My parents reported what was happening to my teachers and eventually two girls were moved to other schools. I was relieved, but one night I was on MSN Messenger and received a death threat. My parents went to the police and eventually we got harassment orders issued against both girls. That meant they couldn't come near me or my family or try to make contact."

In July, the Temple school district in Central Texas added online or cyberbullying to its Code of Student Conduct. According to the code, reports tdtnews.com, "a student can be punished for using someone's name, without their consent, with the intent to "harm, defraud, intimidate, or threaten," according to the language of the section." This is one school district that realizes how important it is to set a precedent to control the behavior of online bullies.

Cyberbullying is a complicated topic, and one that is just starting to be researched. The Internet is hard to regulate because of free speech laws, and because so many of these issues regarding the Internet are so new that we simply have not been able to catch up yet. Eventually, lawmakers will realize that we need to find a way to legislate abuse and aggression perpetuated on the Internet just like we do offline. Until then, we need proactive vigilance and education to learn how to stop cyberbullying in its tracks. Some have been successful suing individual perpetuators but that is not an easy or feasible tact for all. With increased observation and by educating everyone in your community what cyberbullying is, you can be well on your way to stamping it out.

5. Anxiety and Depression

Anxiety. What a dreaded feeling! What an awful emotion! No one likes to have anxiety. No one likes the worrying, the jitters, the all consuming self consciousness, the thoughts in your head that won't stop.

When you have anxiety, you can't enjoy the things around you, you can't even focus on the things around you. You can't feel good about yourself, you can't attend to your friends or classes; you have a million worrisome thoughts running through your head. And depression too often goes with anxiety. When someone has too much anxiety, they can start thinking "What good is it all? What good is trying? Nothing I do will ever come out right. Nothing I do is worth it. I will never be able to do this right. I just know it." This leads to feelings of depression and the person can become very demotivated to even keep trying; they can feel everything is futile. Anxiety and depression, unfortunately, go hand in hand and are very common in teens with Aspergers.

What does anxiety feel like?

The technical definition of anxiety is "A feeling of apprehension and fear characterized by physical symptoms such as palpitations, sweating, and feelings of stress." (med-terms.com) But what does it feel like, especially for the teen with Aspergers? Well, a teen with AS is likely to be worried about many things. "What if the bully in the hallway pushes me again today? What if they don't have turkey sandwiches for lunch? What if I forget or lose my lunch money? What if the teacher calls on me in class? What if she doesn't? What if I have extra questions I need help with? What if the bus is late? What if it rains and I don't have an umbrella to use to go out at lunchtime? What if the noise of all the people in the hallways is too overwhelming? What if I can't finish my paper before the deadline?"

There are so many things to worry about, from the perspective of an AS teen. Obsessive worry, like the examples above, is common in many AS teens. They may seem smart, and they are. You might think that they're smart enough to know not to worry about some of those things. But despite being smart, they don't sometimes have the emotional smarts you might think they do.

Why are AS teens so anxious?

Teens with Aspergers get lost in their emotions and feelings of frustration. Their need to have everything just so, their need for predictability, their need to have some measure of control over what is happening to them can lead to intense anxiety. They may be having social problems and worry that they'll never have friends. Some older teens who have more self-awareness may realize that they're not functioning the same way as their peers and wonder what this will mean once they get out of high school or for later in life. Most are worried about more day to day concerns, though.

Anxiety and school

A school is such an ever-changing environment. Every day, hundreds of kids go in and out; they use the classrooms, bathrooms, athletic fields, and lunch room. With so many people, the variant behavior, the potential for things to go in different ways and be unpredictable, is huge. Even the sensory information is unpredictable and can be over-whelming: lockers banging at random intervals, kids shouting in the hallways, people running, bells being played over the intercom, and so on. For a teen with AS who has sensory issues, the unpredictability of these sounds and events can lead to a lot of anxiety. They know that these things cause distress and they naturally are leery of putting themselves in a situation that causes so much stress.

Six Reasons Why School Anxiety Is A Very Common Problem In Teens With AS

1. Many AS teens have poor motor skills and little interest in sports. Especially for boys, this may isolate them among their peers.

2. Due to quirky behavior, speech patterns or preoccupations with special interests, AS teens are often bullied.

3. Because of their social naiveté, AS teens often get made fun of.

4. The sensory environment can be too much for them.

5. Transitions between classes can be overwhelming.

6. The stress of trying to figure out how to function socially can be too much for them.

What are some symptoms of anxiety? How do you know your kid has it?

Anxiety can show in many, many different ways; it can cause all kinds of physical problems as well as emotional issues and thought distortion. It is important for parents to recognize the signs of anxiety. The following table lists fourteen common signs to look for.

14 Common Symptoms of Anxiety

1. Excessive, ongoing worry and tension
2. An unrealistic view of problems
3. Restlessness or a feeling of being "edgy"
4. Irritability
5. Muscle tension
6. Headaches
7. Sweating
8. Difficulty concentrating
9. Nausea
10. The need to go to the bathroom frequently
11. Tiredness
12. Trouble falling or staying asleep
13. Trembling
14. Being easily startled

Avoidant Behavior

If you're not in your kid's school every day, and they don't talk to you much, or you're not around them enough to observe the above symptoms, how do you know your teen with AS is suffering from anxiety? Well, one way is if they exhibit avoidant behaviors. Do they try to get out of going to school in the morning? Do they cut particular classes? If they're trying to avoid school or certain aspects of it, even if they try to mask this emotion or phrase it in other ways – "I'm bored in that class, it's so easy!" "The teacher doesn't know anything; it's not worth my time!" – then they might be exhibiting problems of a moderate to severe anxiety problem.

Relieving Your Teen's Anxiety

If your teen's anxiety is so bad that it is interfering with his or her ability to attend classes, go to school, understand what they or learning, or be able to function in a normal school or out of school setting, there are several things you can do.

1. Identify the cause of their anxiety

The first thing that is important is to identify what is causing their anxiety. You want to make sure you are addressing the right issues. If it is caused by sensory issues like loud noises in the hall, getting jostled by people walking in between classes, or bullying in the halls, ask the school to work with you to take steps to make sure this does not happen. Arrange for your teen to be able to leave classes five minutes early so that they can have empty hallways to travel in, or get to classes five minutes late. Or perhaps have an aide who can travel with your teen to be a soothing presence and keep bullies at bay – older teens may not want to have the stigma of having an aide, however.

2. Consider a special education classroom

Your teen might feel more comfortable in a self contained classroom, called by several names such as a learning cen-

73

ter, where they can go and get some extra help and attention and be in an environment that is more sensitive to their needs. Usually students who have learning difficulties or other problems will come here for extra help. Teachers are usually more aware of dynamics between students and there are usually fewer students in the classroom. This can be either a drop in center your teen goes to when he or she needs a break, or it can be a special education classroom they go to all day. Even if your teen is smart and can ace all the academic material of their classes, they may be having anxiety about other areas of school life and could benefit from a special education classroom. If you live in a big enough area, there might be classes or services especially for teens with Aspergers.

3. Use social stories to tell them what will happen next

Another big issue is that AS teens worry about what is going to happen next. When they were a small child, you used social stories to tell them what would happen. This might still work for some teens, but for others who have gotten older and "grown out" of them, a modified version will still work. Make a schedule for them and write it out on paper, so they will know everything that will happen in the course of a school day. Include things like what time they will get up in the morning, what they will eat for breakfast, what time they will get to school, how long in each class, what time each class starts and ends and where it is located, what time lunch is, any special pull-outs such as speech or occupational therapy. Go over it with them. Make sure they understand it. And, most importantly, make sure they know what to do if things go wrong.

4. Find your kid a supportive adult

If they get overwhelmed in between classes, or someone makes fun of them, or they just need a time out – identify someone in the school whom they can go to, to talk, to get some support, or just to get a break. Maybe there's a learning center type place, maybe the school office, maybe the counselor's office – make sure they have a person who they can go to for a time out, an escape route. This person can help them calm down or just give them some space. **If your AS teen feels like they have control over things that might go wrong and ways to rectify problems that do come up, they will be a lot more comfortable going to school and being in school.**

5. Home schooling

If your teen's anxiety becomes overwhelming and debilitating, you might want to consider home schooling if that is an option or a special education school that is smaller and better suited to their needs, if you have the means. (In some cases, school districts will pay for this if you can prove that there is no way the school district can adequately meet your needs and provide an equal education.)

What causes depression in teens with Aspergers?

Depression, like most things, is measured by degree. Everyone has days where they feel a little blue or a little out of sorts; where they are little more irritable and pessimistic than usual. But it is when once in a while turns into almost every day, and the feeling grow in intensity until you can't think of anything but how bad you feel, that you have a problem.

> ➢ **Anxiety**

Anxiety can lead to depression for teens with Aspergers, as I said above. The feeling of getting up everyday dreading the day and worrying about what will happen can take a toll on you after a while. If the anxiety is preventing you from participating in activities you would otherwise engage in, you might start getting a negative opinion of yourself. You might start to think you're not able to do the things you need to do.

Aspergers teens may have so much anxiety that they cannot participate in classes, after school activities, make friends, date, or do the usual things kids their age do. They have negative thoughts. They might start feeling worthless.

"I can't make any friends."

"People seem to hate me no matter what I do."

"People think I'm weird."

"I can't understand what my teachers are saying."

"I can't get my homework done. I must be a failure at life."

This kind of thinking can be deadly, of course. After a while, all they want to do is sleep, or go on the computer, or play video games – mind numbing activities that keep them from experiencing the pain of life. They may cry a lot, become very irritable, snap at people, or just completely withdraw and do nothing. They may refuse to take part in activities outside of the house.

> **Isolation**

Feelings of isolation can also lead to depression. Repeated social failures at school, bullying, a lack of a feeling of connection to others, even if the teen appears to have friends (who may only be very superficial friends or may be teasing your teen without you knowing it), can lead to feelings of depression. If your teen is very smart but doesn't have many friends, they may be frustrated that there is no one on their intellectual level that they can share things with or discuss ideas. If they have unusual interests, they may be lonely without anyone to share them with.

What are other symptoms of depression?

Like anxiety, depression can manifest in many different ways. Depression can lead to serious problems such as drug abuse, problems at school, low self esteem, self injury, reckless behavior and even suicide. It is important for parents and school officials to recognize the signs and symptoms of depression because many teenagers will not directly seek help for depression until it is too late. The following table lists the most common symptoms of depression in teenagers:

12 Common Symptoms of Depression in Teenagers

1. Sadness or hopelessness

2. Irritability, anger, or hostility

3. Tearfulness or frequent crying

4. Withdrawal from friends and family

5. Loss of interest in activities

6. Changes in eating and sleeping habits

7. Restlessness and agitation

8. Feelings of worthlessness and guilt

9. Lack of enthusiasm and motivation

10. Fatigue or lack of energy

11. Difficulty concentrating

12. Thoughts of death or suicide

What can I do if my AS teen seems depressed?

1. Communicate and support

It is important to maintain lines of communication with your teenager so you can assess whatever problems they may be having, and be a source of support that they can turn to when they need it. Try to offer support to your teen without being too pushy or intrusive. Try to just listen without judging. Don't ask a lot of questions. Just be there for them. Also, be gentle, but keep trying; continually make it clear to your teen that you are there to listen to them and help them in whatever way they need. Try to validate their feelings, and try to avoid giving any lectures about what they should or should not do. These tips will help your teen feel more comfortable coming to you when they need to talk, and hopefully lessen the feelings of depression and isolation.

2. Have your teen join a special interest group

Do anything you can think of to give your teen a sense of meaning, purpose, and inclusion. Find groups that your teen can be a part of and social activities that they can take part in. This may be a group of other teens who have social challenges that your teen can be a part of. Many AS teens have special interests – find a group of link-minded individuals who have formed a special interest group or club. This may be on chess, or computers, or any number of areas where your teenager has an interest and will feel a part of something. Talk to your school counselor or local autism resource groups, or other parents, to find these things. A useful resource is to use *www.meetup.com*. This is a web site that lists, by area, meetings of like minded people. Just type in a subject (like stamp collecting or Aspergers support groups) then type in your city and country and any group that is registered will be listed. I have used this web site many times to help others find Aspergers support groups in their areas.

3. Create a task where your teen can succeed

You can also make up tasks and chores for them to do that will not be too overwhelming. Perhaps a bedroom needs painting or a fence needs some repair. Or simply wash or wax a car. Pick a task that shows visible results when your teen is finished. Make a big deal of the accomplishment and let it be a symbol of success that your teen can be proud of.

4. Give lots of praise

Play up their good points and strengths. Give them lots of praise. Talk to them about the meaning of difference, and how just because they do things differently, think differently, and communicate differently, they are just as good as their peers, and will go just as far in life; they just need to do it a little bit differently and might need a little support in some areas to succeed. Talk about people like Einstein and Bill Gates who had social difficulties but still made real contributions to the world.

Therapy and Medication

When your teen's feelings of anxiety or depression become too large to be managed by any of the strategies I have described above, that's when you need to seek outside help.

➤ **Therapy**

Therapy and counseling can help greatly; it can give the teen with Aspergers a safe, neutral place where they feel like their feelings, worries and concerns are being heard. Where they can feel validated. Counselors can teach better social skills and how to handle your emotions; they can teach coping skills for how to handle the stress of everyday life, plus the special issues and challenges that come along with Aspergers. They can give your teen more perspective on their challenges, and be an encouraging voice. It's best to find a therapist versed in Aspergers, but anyone your teen feels a connection with will do. Different types of therapies that are available will be discussed in a later chapter.

➢ Medications

Additionally, there are many medications on the market today that have been proven to help with anxiety and depression. There are anti-depressant medicines, called SSRIs, like Prozac that can help with depression; there are anti-anxiety medications like Ativan and Valium; even some types of anti-psychotic and off label uses of anti-seizure medications have shown to be helpful in reducing anxiety in people with Aspergers so they can have more functioning in their daily life.

A good psychiatrist will be able to tell you what they think is the best choice for your teen's symptoms. The different classes of medications will be reviewed more thoroughly in a later chapter.

When Should I Tell My Kid They Have Aspergers?

I include this section in the chapter on anxiety and depression because not knowing what's wrong with you or what makes you so different from others can be a huge source of both anxiety and depression, especially when you get to be a teenager.

Many parents wonder, when should I let my kid know what they have? Is it placing too much of a burden on them to give them this label? Will I encourage them to act out more or give them an excuse if they know they have disorder? Will they understand what I mean? Will a label detract from what they are able to do, will it "mark" them in a negative way?

These are all arguments, of course, for not telling your child about Aspergers. I personally don't think any of them are valid. You should tell your child about Aspergers as soon as you know – in an age-appropriate way. Your child is going to know they are different no matter what you do. Their peers will make it clear to them that they don't fit in, that there is something off. Kids, and teens, are sensitive to this kind of information and will realize even if you don't think they are aware of it. They might not share their feelings of being different with you because they are trying to protect you, or are afraid of your reaction.

The sooner that a person with Aspergers can learn what Aspergers is, how it makes them different, why it makes them different, and how they can learn coping strategies to get around their differences, the better off they will be in life. The sooner they can learn to accept themselves, and learn that different is not a disease, that they are fine just the way they are, but will need to work harder in certain areas to make up for certain weaknesses, the better off they will be. They will be more confident and much less likely to fall into depression or anxiety if they are well-grounded and have a good sense of who they are – both their positive traits and their negative ones.

For parents of small kids, you might not want to call it by its name as that could be too confusing and overwhelming. You might just want to say "You have some parts of you that are very sensitive and get overwhelmed easily. We love you and we want to help you with these parts of you. That's why we're taking you to therapy to help you, or why you sometimes get frustrated," or so on. Depending on the child, once they get into perhaps fourth or fifth grade, you can give it a name – because everyone else will, so you might as well give them the correct name. You know your child's level of maturity and intelligence better than anyone, so you can judge how much to tell at what time. The general rule of thumb, though, is more is better, and always **take care to phrase what you are saying in a positive way and talk to your child about their positive traits** so they will see this is not something to be depressed about or worry about too much.

If you do this, by the time your child is a teenager, they will have a good sense of who they are, and will be much better able to advocate for themselves and their needs, and to stand up to bullies who try to put them down because they are different. So, by all means, if you haven't told your child they have Aspergers by the time they enter high school, do so now. Knowing WHY you are different, and having a name for it, is a huge part of self esteem for kids in this age group. Most young adults surveyed as to whether or not they want to know what they have, have said they definitely do want to know and that finding out came as a big relief. Most young adults who don't get diagnosed till their 20s or later are glad to have a label to their difference and wish they had known earlier, particularly in their school years.

It is not too late, however, if you neglected to give this information earlier; just keep working on playing up the positive parts and let your teen vent to you about the negatives when they are having a hard time.

Anxiety and Depression from the Eyes of a Teenager with Aspergers

It is one thing to talk about and discuss what anxiety and depression are, what they feel like, and how they manifest in teenagers with Aspergers, but it is even better to learn from an actual teenager with Aspergers how these things feel to her. We can gain a better sense of understanding about the issues our kids struggle with by reading about others who have been here.

Printed with the permission of a 17 year old with Aspergers is a thoughtful essay on anxiety, social connection, difference and the meaning of life. We can see her feelings of depression about not measuring up to her peers, anxiety about where her life is going to lead and worries about whether she will ever get the social connection and friends she so much desires. These are some of the key issues to address for teens with Aspergers.

> Reflections on Human Connection and the Meaning of Life
>
> How do you know when you have truly made a connection with someone, when you have a true friendship, as opposed to people just acting friendly? Not that I don't love friendly people and carrying on small talk with them just for the sake of talking to someone, because I do, but my heart yearns for more than that. I want to be with people, I want to have all the friends I never had when I was a kid growing up, I want to experience the social side of life. I have no idea what that would be like but it feels like it is the missing ingredient in my life – junk food is great but can only take you so far and I am seriously worried for the quality of my life if the only thing that can make me happy is food. I am glad food can make me happy just the same but it would be very nice to have more than that.

I was thinking earlier about how you know you have a connection with someone while talking to two of my aunts on the phone. Well, I called one and had a long conversation with her, and then almost as soon as I had hung up, my other aunt on the opposite side of the country called. I realized after I talked to my second aunt that maybe this was what connection was. It is talking to someone and having time stop while you're doing that, it is being able to bask in the warmth and comfort of their voice, it is not being scared while you are talking to them, it is a feeling of immunity against all that normally troubles you while you are with them. It is a feeling of hope and a feeling that something in your heart is being temporarily filled up. The missing piece is, for a precious few minutes, there again. It is feeling good about yourself, feeling more in sync with the universe, feeling you matter. Feeling worth in yourself. It cuts through the loneliness like a knife.

That is what a good conversation can do. That is why I crave connections with people so much. But the feeling is alas only temporary. Almost as soon as I hang up or leave the person the feeling of loneliness and of being cut off and isolated comes over me again. Maybe I am happy for several minutes, as I frantically try to go over every word of the conversation in my head and commit it to memory and try as hard as I can, always in vain but never lacking in effort, to get it through my thick skull that it is possible to feel connected to people, to store the memory in my heart for later times when I will need it.

I have a diary going back two or three years of these moments in an effort to prove to myself that I have something to live for. And it's really discouraging to me that after all this effort, I still find myself feeling basically disconnected and unsatisfied with life. That I find myself, with some change in degree but not nearly enough, just about as lonely , isolated and desperate as I was several years ago. Things are supposed to change in all that time, aren't they? It's astounding to me sometimes. I have made a few more friends, I am little more comfortable socially, I have accepted to a greater degree my outsider status and am a little more comfortable with myself – but it's not nearly enough. I'm still on the outside.

At school my feelings of social isolation are more painful and intense because I'm constantly surrounded by people my age who I compare myself to constantly. I never feel good enough around them. It makes me feel rather depressed more than I would like.

I treasure every word, though. Every word of every good conversation I have with anyone. The conversations in the computer lab, the conversations with the librarians, every interaction with a teacher that I like, every bit of small talk waged with a classmate, the occasional encounters when someone actually comes up to me to start a conversation (that usually started with "What are you listening to?", referring to my always present Walkman. Every conversation with a teacher. Not that it isn't hard — I walk back and forth in the halls of the school for ten, twenty minutes, trying to get the nerve to knock on a teacher's door, fighting the feelings of insecurity and anxiety and fear when I start conversations with people, trying to figure out what to say and how long the conversation should go on for and what I can possibly do to make myself appear more acceptable. The self hatred and loneliness as I watch others interact so easily and be surrounded by so many friends, that is always present. Trying to break through those feelings to make an effort to connect with people so I can kill those feelings of loneliness.

The wonderful back and forth of a conversation — how many people do you know who simply treasure being part of a conversation? Well, I should be more specific here. I don't enjoy arguments, shouting fests, anything tense or unpredictable. I don't enjoy talking to uncommunicative or unfriendly people. But I thrive on friendly, open, warm people. Conversation with them is like a miraculous game of ping pong, where the ball goes back and forth and I am amazed that I am able to keep it in motion. It doesn't matter so much what we talk about, but I treasure the warmth in their voice, the smile on their face, the brief sense of connection. I soak up this feeling of connection.

Yet, these are crumbs, mere crumbs, and how long can a person exist on mere crumbs? What is there to say it will ever change in the future and why should I live a life doomed to the kind of isolation and desperation I have felt and struggled boldly with all my life? There needs to be a reason, that's all I can say.

Without a purpose in life, without something to do with my time, my life, my intellect, without a way to connect and be with others, without a way to make meaning in my life, I am just whittling away the days on the calendar, and I cannot stand that. I don't like to think about it, but it is the truth. The truth is I spend all my time looking for ways to kill time and for things to do where I can not be thinking about the truth of my life.

I have things to offer the world. I am aware enough to realize that. I have a sense of humor, a positive and up-beat personality when I can possibly manage it, infectious enthusiasm again whenever I can, a gentle personality that genuinely cares about people and aims to help them whenever I can. I am intelligent and analytical. I am loyal and try hard at whatever I do...for the most part. There is so much I want to experience in the world. It wouldn't take much to make me happy – just feeling like I was part of something would be enough. Just feeling like I mattered, like I had some purpose no matter how small. Just having a friend or two, a real friend. It wouldn't take much.

I am frustrated to realize that if I didn't have some of the difficulties that I have due to my Aspergers, that I might have the potential to be a very satisfied person and to be able to give something of myself and make a difference to the world. Instead, I just feel overwhelmed and tossed about and unable to function in the way I want to function. I feel like my life is a long battle that unfortunately won't end any time soon. I don't like it.

Anonymous

***

Again, this poignant essay describes many of the key themes that teenagers with Aspergers often deal with. They try as hard as they can, but often find that they just can't connect with people in the way they want to. They don't have the words, the nuances, the skills to be able to connect. Their intelligence, considered an asset by many adults, just sets them apart more and makes it harder for them to find similar people who they can connect with. Their differences make them a target for bullies, which lowers their self-esteem and makes them more prone to anxiety and depression.

Even if bullying is not an issue, or was an issue but has stopped, the self-comparison teens often do of themselves to others can be quite destructive. Not all teens with Aspergers are going to be exactly like this writer in how much social contact they want or in what ways they go about to get it, but the themes of anxiety, depression and not being good enough are universal. Again, we need programs in our schools that can help our kids with Aspergers to realize the strengths they have, and to be able to look at themselves and their challenges in a more positive light. This is especially important in getting our kids through their teenage years as unscathed as possible.

6. Social Issues: Making Friends and Building Relationships

Think for a minute, if you will, about what gets you through each day. Is it knowing that you have someone who understands you that you can tell your troubles to when the day is over? Is it looking forward to that friend you can shoot the breeze with when your time at the office is up? Is it the connection you feel with your friends that gives you strength, energy and support to face one more day in this hectic, fast paced world we live in?

Our sense of community and our connections to other people are a very important factor in how we live. Just knowing that other people are going through similar things, and being able to laugh it off at the end of the day, is a very powerful motivating factor. Developers spend millions to build neighborhoods with some kind of center where people can gather; at college campuses, clubs and group activities flourish; people seem to take every opportunity they can to get together.

Friends, then, you might agree, are a very important part of life. They strengthen us; they give us someone to lean on when we need a boost; they make us laugh; they give us a feeling of connection, a feeling of belonging; they contribute to our mental health.

Problems Making Friends

But for teens with Asperger's Syndrome, friends can some-times seem like the seventh class on their already packed high school schedule. One more thing to learn; one more thing to figure out; one more thing that just doesn't make any sense.

Because teens with AS have such difficulty reading social cues, they can't seem to pick up on the "social slang" that many teens use; they can't talk easily and casually like so many teens do. Because of this, they are often shunned. They can't break into conversations. They stand just on the outside, looking in.

Many teens with AS wants friends but can't figure out how to get them; some don't have any desire for them. For those who want them but can't figure out how to make friends, it can be especially painful. They try the best they know how; they talk about spaceships and current events and politics. Topics that make sense to them. They don't know that these topics don't interest their peers. They might try to copy their friends' language and words but it comes out sounding forced and scripted. Most of their peers just don't have the patience for their oddity and awkwardness.

UCLA psychiatry instructor Elizabeth Laugeson commented on why it is so difficult for teens with Asperger's to make friends in a recent study on the topic (http://a4.org.au/a4/node/83).

> "'It's hard enough to be a teenager," she said, "but it's harder still for adolescents with autism because they typically lack the ability to pick up on all the social cues most of us take for granted – things like body language, hand gestures and facial expres-sions, along with speech inflections like warmth, sarcasm or hostility.

"Lack of these basic social skills may lead to rejection, isolation or bullying from their peers. And sadly, that isolation can carry into their adult life.

How do you have a successful get-together with someone? How do you go up to a group of teens and join their conversation? What do you say as a comeback when someone teases you? Without these core social skills, it becomes very difficult for teenagers to make and keep friends," Laugeson said."

Reasons Teens with Asperger's Have Trouble Making Friends

Wanting friends is one thing, but making them and keeping them is another entirely. Intelligence has nothing to do with it. You need a certain social savvy to make friends that most teens with AS lack.

Some particular things that can get the Asperger's teen in trouble are:

1. Odd mannerisms

AS teens often talk too loudly, can't modulate their tone of voice, might interrupt others without realizing it, might avoid eye contact, might violate the physical space of others without being aware, and might talk too much about their favorite topic.

Some Aspie teens have a hard time sharing their thoughts and opinions, and this can make them seem aloof and standoffish.

Because of anxiety from past negative experiences and just the difficulty of it all, most Aspie teens are reluctant to initiate social interaction with others, and few teens, with the exception of unusually kind and insightful teens, will initiate contact with them.

2. Rule oriented

Many Aspie teens are very rule oriented and this doesn't work very well in a teenage population where everyone is all about defying, bending and ignoring every rule possible. Most teens don't want to be told what to do and don't want to follow a schedule; but most Aspie teens can't bear to do anything without having a schedule and planning everything out ahead of time

3. Ignorance of Teen Culture

Most Aspie teens are not aware of the latest clothing trends and styles; they may not be aware of how they're dressing; their hygiene may be lacking. Most typical teens are obsessed with how they look and Aspie teens that don't think about this often have a hard time fitting in.

4. Immature interests

Often Aspie teens will have interests left over from elementary school; they may be interested in games, fads, or TV shows that passed by long ago. This is another thing that makes it hard for them to connect with their peers.

5. Sensory issues

Everything is too loud, too fast, too bright, too confusing to the teen with Asperger's who also has sensory issues. AS teens often don't like bowling alleys with loud music, loud restraints, or any place crowded. They get overwhelmed very easily by their environment. This is another challenge for doing things with friends and can create a lot of difficulty.

Problems can lead to isolation

Problems making friends can lead to social isolation, depression, and high anxiety for teens with AS. They may become hopeless, thinking that no one will ever like them, that life is not worth living. They may rebel and get into dangerous behavior such as drugs, drinking, or trouble with the law. They may withdraw, or be subjected to bullying which further damages their self-esteem.

Not all teens with Asperger's will have this much trouble with friends. Some will find other kids that also don't fit in well and make friends with them. Some will struggle but ultimately find those other kids who have enough patience to understand them. Some just don't seem to care or suffer from lack of friends; they're happy on their own. But for those teens who want nothing more than to go to Dairy Queen on Saturday night with a couple of buddies, go to a baseball game or fishing, or do girl talk, it can feel devastating not to have friends.

How To Help Teens with Asperger's Make Friends

How, then, can we try to fix this problem? How can we give people on the autistic spectrum a sense of community, a sense of connection and break through their isolation? Fortunately, there has been much research done and many tried and true methods to help Aspie teens make friends. Not all will work for everyone; but some will usually work for most everyone, given the right kind of support and enough time.

1. Interest groups

The easiest way to help Aspie teens make friends is to find out what they're interested in, and find a group of teens who are interested in the same thing. If all goes well, their shared interest in a topic will overcome any social awkwardness; the Aspie teen will hopefully feel more comfortable discussing a topic of interest. Groups that are slightly "geeky" or intellectual in nature may have a better chance of containing members that will better be able to get along with your Aspie teen.

A great place to find groups is to use www.meetup.com. You can type in your country and city (or in the U.S., your zip code). Then type in a topic of interest (fishing, rock collecting, trains – you name it) and it will list any clubs/groups in your area. I have used it to find Aspergers support groups in my area.

2. Mentors

Many schools have peer mentoring programs; these are usually staffed by kids more likely to be kind, sensitive, and understanding to differences. They might be able to help your teen strike up a friendship. Or else try to use a university student as a mentor, for the same reason; more maturity, and if they work one-on-one with your teen, your teen will flourish in the attention and care of someone older. It will help to raise their self esteem and give them the courage to try to approach their peers.

3. Help plan activities

Help your teen identify activities that their peers may be interested in. This could be going to a movie or watching one at home; having a pizza night; playing video games; going to a mini golf course; biking; anything that they can think of. Help your teen set up the activity and help them figure who to invite and how to invite a few peers for a night of fun. Discuss ahead of time things to talk about and appropriate behavior.

4. Social skills groups

Find social skills groups in your area, run by qualified counselors. They can help your teen learn things like social cues, social skills, and how to be more aware of the way they are coming across. They can help Aspie teens to pick up on signs of interest from peers. Social groups give Aspie teens a safe place to practice their social skills before they try them out on peers at school.

Here is a good site that may help you find a social skills group in your area:

www.asperger.org/Prof_and_Parent_Support.asp

5. Find local Asperger's support groups in your area

There are many support groups for teens with Asperger's. Sometimes, it is easier to try to make friends with others who have the same neurological difference that you. They understand you without you having to explain. They don't judge. You can speak the same language. Many Aspie teens find it an enormous relief to be with other Aspies and find that they can make friends and be social for the first time.

More information on how to find local Asperger's support groups for your teen

Finding other socially awkward people can be one of the best bets for your teen to be able to connect with another person. It just works better when you are coming from the same background. There are many ways to find other Aspies to connect with, both online and off. Here are some of them.

Online Support for Teens with Asperger's

Internet Aspie communities can be divided into several different groups. First, there are the message boards. Users converge on message boards and talk about every aspect of their lives possible. The biggest of these sites is www.WrongPlanet.net. www.WrongPlanet.net currently has over eight thousand members registered from all over the world.

The beauty of online Aspie message boards is that the anonymity and the medium makes it much easier to communicate. Most Aspies have a much easier time writing their thoughts rather than speaking them and therefore, benefit enormously from online Aspie communities. People talk about their interests, rehash social situations that may not have gone so well and ask for advice about them, talk about medical problems, and ask advice about everything you can imagine. They gain support from knowing they are not alone, from knowing other people are experiencing the same things they are.

WrongPlanet.net is split into sections like General Autism Discussion, Love and Dating, Friendship and General Social Interaction, the Haven (for sensitive issues), School and College Life, and Work and Finding a Job. There are forums for people's interests, for getting to know each other, for adult issues, and for women. A current sampling of topics on Wrong Planet at this writing are topics such as childhood fears, Asperger's resources in San Francisco, problems talking on the phone, crying in public, depression, feeling like an outcast, and whether or not tell your manager at work that you have AS.

Online discussion groups can give you practical advice and emotional support, and occasionally you even find someone who lives in your area who can become a friend offline as well as online.

There are also email groups, the most popular of these being Yahoo groups [groups.yahoo.com]. With a Yahoo email group, you subscribe to a particular group and get emails from other people who have also subscribed. You can read their messages and reply. There are an abundance of Yahoo groups on autism spectrum issues – one needs to only search their website for "autism" or "aspergers" to find them.

Offline Support Groups for Teens with Asperger's

There exist several national AS organizations with local chapters that might be able to help.

There is an organization based in Boston called Asperger's Association of New England [www.aane.org] that runs support groups for adults with AS all throughout New England. In Boston, they not only have the usual monthly support groups, but they also have discussion groups, social activity groups, movie nights and all kinds of other activities for adults with AS.

In New York, there is an organization called GRASP [www.grasp.org], or the Global Regional Aspergers Partnership. GRASP runs support groups for adults in several different states. They have groups in New York, Long Island, Philadelphia, Virginia Beach, Denver, and other cities. Each GRASP network is independently run by someone in one of those cities who decides they want to undertake it, and gets support and guidance from the New York organization. GRASP even runs a separate group for Orthodox Jewish people in New York. GRASP runs a group for teens in the New York City area.

Local groups can be found in your area by contacting school counselors, local therapists, or other moms with kids with Asperger's.

Many groups are run by local therapists or other clinicians for teens with Asperger's. Your local branch of the Autism Society of America [www.autism-society.org] might know of some groups in your area. Or, if you can't find one already there - start your own! Run an ad in the paper or ask the school therapist for help. Also, search Google for local groups in your area.

One young adult, on writing about her experience of meeting others with Asperger's, had this to say about the importance of Aspies meeting other Aspies for friendship:

"As Aspies, all our lives the only message we have been able to consistently pick up on from the people around us was that we were doing something wrong. We were always doing something wrong, almost every minute of the day it seemed sometimes, but we could never figure out what. We could not connect with the people around us; we were afraid of them and could not understand them. Now, years later in a room full of Aspies, we can start to relearn some of the messages told to us. We can start to replace "You're wrong/weird/awkward/socially deficient" with "You're articulate/interesting/knowledgeable/passionate/just like me!" We can start to realize that there really is nothing wrong with the way we communicate, that other people share our interests, other people share our seemingly bizarre single minded passions, our literal mindedness, our attention to details, even our naiveté. We can start to see these things as good things instead of bad and different. It is like a "re-enculturation" process: we are learning the norms of a culture (Aspie culture) that finally allows us to define ourselves as good, competent people."

We can see then, that it is so important for our Asperger's teens to be able to make friends, whether with quirky typical peers or with other Asperger's teens.

PERSPECTIVE FROM A YOUNG WOMAN WITH ASPERGER'S

I want to close this section on Asperger's teens and friends by including further insight by a young woman with Asperger's on her struggles with friendship over the years. As I've said in previous chapters, we can learn so much about what Asperger's is like for our kids by reading the words of those who have lived it. We can learn from the struggles of others and start to understand the experience. This can motivate us to find ways around these struggles to make a better experience for our kids.

***

"I remember only a few teasing incidents from these years, strangely enough. There must have been more to have created such a strong sense of fear and otherness from people – or maybe that was always there, a result of my Asperger's, who knows? I often wonder – but I can only remember a few incidents. I know I wrote in my diary about people who were mean to me or who tried to steal my stuff, but it was nothing compared with what happened to me in later years. So why I was so traumatized, I don't know. But it was just the way I was.

And I didn't realize I was, didn't know I was, obviously couldn't put any words to it – it was the only thing I had ever known, the only way I had ever felt, how could I know it was different? All I knew was the feeling of wanting to be away from people, or at least people my own age (I seemed to get along well with babysitters, parents well enough, and some teachers). I couldn't relate to my peers in the least. I spent my time reading, writing, and playing endless board games with my babysitters. As well as just getting lost in my own head.

Speaking of that, that was another coping mechanism I had. Getting lost in my own head. I developed the most complex and intricate games to play in my head whenever I had any downtime. I remember being on the school bus and playing "Guess how many kids will be at the next stop" or playing the ABC game – I would try to make sentences where each word started with the same letter of the alphabet, starting from Anna Ate An Apple all the way to X, Y and Z. I had a complex scoring and point system based on the number of letters used in each word and the length of each sentence. I had several similar word games I played in my head. I played them constantly whenever I was in a scary, unfamiliar or boring situation; I needed to occupy my thoughts and feelings to numb the pain of the outside world, I think. Funny thing is I don't remember labeling it as such; I don't remember ever thinking "I'm sad," "I'm in pain," or any such thing other than "I'm scared," but even then I didn't really label it as such as much as feel it and act in ways to try to mediate it or get away from it (reading, games in my head, staying away from other kids).

I did well in school academically. I followed directions. I was a good and compliant student. I participated in all mandatory activities, like plays and such. But I did it all from a million miles away. I didn't feel connected to anyone. I just felt this all encompassing sense of, when with adults, "What do I have to do to make this person like me/not be mad at me" and with kids "What do I have to do to make them be nice to me." Or, more often "How soon can I get away from them?"

The thing is, despite all this anxiety and fear that came so naturally, I didn't even realize that I didn't have friends until the start of junior high. The concept had never really occurred to me! It would be like someone asking me "Do you want to go to the moon," that's how relevant having friends seemed.

When I entered seventh grade, then, I was just starting to awaken to the realization of what friends were. It was like I was becoming awake and aware to the world for the first time. For the first time, I noticed other kids doing things together. I noticed how kids were always in pairs, talking. I noticed laughing and groups of kids. And I began to think "Wait, why aren't I like that? I want to be in a pair like that, and have someone to do stuff with. How do I get that?" I began to realize what a friend was, and realize I wanted one. But I had NO idea, not the slightest idea, how to go about getting one. Thus ensued three years of depression and eventually suicidal idealization as I for the first time in my life realized how different I was, and had no explanation for it.

Eighth grade was my hell on earth year; it was a year full of intense bullying, both physical and verbal; I won't go into specifics. It was constant and never ending, and mostly done by the same two guys. I was extremely scarred by it and what little of my self esteem I had went out the window. But, still, I never labeled it as wrong; I never told anyone; it never occurred to me that it was wrong. I hadn't ever known anything else. I didn't like it, sure, but I didn't know that it was wrong. I didn't know that I deserved more, that it could maybe be stopped. How sad is that? I'd go home and lie on the floor and cry for hours on end. I'd think about suicide, but never seriously, just kind of in the way that someone imagines a vacation they'd like to take but know they never will.

It was a hellish year, but it did end eventually. When ninth grade came around, I was withdrawn, isolated and depressed – and more scared than ever. The bullying had almost completely stopped, but in my mind it hadn't. I was scared of everything. I had a Walkman at that point and listened to the oldies station at every waking moment to drown out other people and my anxiety and fear. It worked, quite well.

Sophomore year of high school gave me my first real friend. She took notice of me and started talking to me in homeroom or between classes. Just a few words or a "How are you," but they made all the difference in the world to me.

The first time she came over to my house was excruciating. I liked her and I wanted to be her friend, but I had NO IDEA what to do with her! I couldn't fathom what friends did together. Talking was so much work. We had nothing real in common. I didn't have the interests that most people my age had. I wasn't into popular culture. I remember sitting in my room thinking "It's only been five minutes, but it feels so LONG."

The one thing we had in common though was a love of music. And even though I liked oldies and she liked country, it was okay. We'd listen to each other's music. We could talk about that. Eventually, she got me from being a steadfast oldies fan to a diehard country fan, but that's another story. She would coax me to listen to these songs, promising I'd like them, and I remember being amazed when I actually did. Maybe even more than her, sometimes. We'd get together and have sleepovers at my house and talk about everything and nothing; and eventually I started to feel close to her.

I am thankful beyond belief that she showed me what it meant to have a friend, she let me feel what it meant to have a friend, she let me experience this thing that in many ways was my saving grace and my social awakening.

The summer before junior year, I went to a sleep-away summer camp for three weeks at Amherst College. The students were all chosen by application process so had a maturity level and intelligence higher than any I'd ever encountered. I begged my mom screaming and crying not to make me go to this camp. I couldn't imagine living with other kids, being alone with other kids, for three weeks. But something amazing happened when I got there. People said hi to me. People talked to me. People actually seemed interested in me. They said I was funny; smart; nice; they wanted to be around me. They LISTENED to me. No one made fun of me. No one even seemed to be in the least mocking me. It was a revelation. Those three weeks were probably the happiest of my life, because I had never felt so included in my life.....before or probably since. I walked to town with other kids; I had conversations with them; sat with them at meals. I didn't even care what we talked about, so happy was I to just be talking to someone.

When I got back to school the next year, I was a changed person. I said hello to every single person I saw in the halls. I talked to kids and teachers alike. I didn't care what I talked about, again, as long as I was talking to people. I made some casual friends who seemed a bit quirky and a bit different from my math class; we hung around in the cafeteria after school and during study hall and talked and even laughed together. Those friendships sustained me and started to teach me what friendship could be like for the first time in my life."

***

In this chapter so far, we have talked about why friendship is important; why teens with Asperger's have such diffi-culty with making friends; how to help them make friends; and we have witnessed a personal account from a young woman with Asperger's and her journey to make friends. Through all this information, we can be more aware of the struggles that our teens with Asperger's face in making friends, and find ways to help them. Everyone deserves to have friends. Asperger's is no reason to give up on the joys of mutual connection. We can change that, together.

Building Relationships with the Opposite Sex

Dating, the other part of the social equation. If teens with Asperger's have trouble making friends, it also goes without saying they have trouble figuring out how to get by in the dating world, too.

At age 13 and on up, most teens are just figuring out what they find desirable in the opposite (or sometimes same) sex. They are figuring out how to court the object of their attraction, how to flirt, what you do on a date, and even how to kiss. This is all immensely exciting to them. Their hormones are going wild and all they can talk about and think about is who's hot and who's not, and who they went out with last night.

Teens with Asperger's want part of this action, too. They also want to talk about who's hot and who they desire. They want to experience the thrill of a goodnight kiss and go on dates as well. But they have several challenges and impediments standing in their way.

Aspie teens often don't know what is socially appropriate and how to communicate their affection for others in an appropriate way.

Guys may appear obsessive in their interest in girls; they may call a girl they like obsessively, catcall her, hound her, try to talk to her constantly. Their behavior can seem almost stalkerish. They are not aware that there is anything wrong in what they are doing. They scare the young girl away.

Girls often don't know how to approach guys, what to say. They are awkward and clumsy. They don't understand social cues or nuance. Both guys and girls have this problem; they turn off who they are trying to attract by not knowing the social rules of dating and flirting. They can't get anyone who they are interested in, interested back.

They may have different ideas of what constitutes a date than their peers do. Guys may try to move too fast without being aware of what the girl wants. Often they just aren't on the same page. It's a problem of first having enough social skills to get noticed, and then having enough social skills to be able to have a successful date. Understanding the difference between friendship and dating, understanding how far to go when, understanding how to have boundaries and set boundaries.

Girls with AS might often get taken advantage of because they don't know how to set boundaries. They don't know what behavior is okay or not for a guy to do to them. They might think they need to do whatever the guy wants to be liked. They need to be taught what is appropriate and how to recognize abuse if and when it is happening.

Aspie teens might feel pressured into having sex too early if they are in a relationship because they feel like they want to keep up with their peers. You should have detailed and explicit conversations with your teen if you think they are going to be engage in this behavior. Share with them the risks and reality of having sex early.

It is important to mention that not ALL teens with Asperger's have an interest in dating. Some prefer not to get involved or just don't have any interest. That is a perfectly valid way to be as well.

How can we help Aspie teens navigate the dating world?

The answer to this is similar to how we would help our teens make friends. Teach them the social skills they will need to learn. Model them. Role play them. Social skills classes, again, can be helpful in this. Peer mentors can be helpful. Creating a list of "rules" for dating, as best you can, can be helpful. You can teach your teen as best you can about how to gauge interest in another person, how to space out calls and interaction to respect the other's space, how to advocate for themselves and set personal boundaries. Above all, just give it time; often Aspie teens acquire the skills needed to figure out the dating world at a later age than their peers. Some will always struggle with this issue, of course, but others will find their way. People with Asperger's do get married and have successful relationships; it just takes some longer than others.

Luke Jackson's book "Freaks, Geeks and Asperger's Syndrome" is a great resource for information on AS teens and dating. Michael John Carley's "Asperger's from the Inside Out" addresses it as well. There are several books that are helpful on this topic and explore it further.

Some Aspies use dating sites to help them find potential matches. Since many people with Asperger's communicate better in writing than in person, online dating sites can level the playing field a little for those with AS. Potential matches can get to know the person with AS, their interests and thoughts and communication style, before they can be distracted by physical things like lack of eye contact, lack of awareness of personal space, and the awkwardness that often shows up more in person. They can get to know the good in the Aspie first.

Dating can be a difficult issue, both for teens and parents. This is true of typical teens as well but it is even more true for teens with Asperger's. Asperger's support groups can be a good place to get advice, help and role modeling for this issue. Teens can share experiences and tell each other what works. Parents should keep an eye on what their teen is doing and offer advice and modeling when possible. Dating is a difficult world to explore, but with a little help, it is possible to be successful in it.

Final Remarks

Friendships and dating are both two very important parts of the social world of the Asperger's teen. Problems with reading social cues and understanding appropriate social behavior can hinder the Asperger's teens in both areas, but peer support, social skills groups, therapists, and parents can help guide the teen with Asperger's in the right direction. Both of these worlds can be navigated by those with Asperger's. An Aspie teen deserves friends and to be able to participate in the dating world just like their typical peers; with a little work, it can happen.

Section Two – Life Beyond High School

So, you have almost finished the hard part: you've almost gotten your teen with Asperger's all the way through high school. All of the IEP meetings, social skills classes, late night homework, and struggles of every day school life will soon stop. Great. But what do you do next? How do you go from the routinized, every minute scheduled life of school to ... anything else?

How do you know if your teen with Asperger's can handle college, and if so, can he handle going away to college or does he need to stay locally? If college isn't in the cards, then what? A job? Will he need a sheltered workshop and lots of support? Can he ever live alone? Will he be eligible for any benefits or support from the government? There are so many questions to answer, when you try to plan for what your teen will do after high school ends. This chapter will try to answer most of them.

7. How to Succeed with Asperger's in the Workplace

You may worry that your teen will never be able to find a workplace that he can fit into; that they will never be able to develop marketable skills. But don't worry, lack of success in high school is not equal to lack of success in the workplace for many with Asperger's. The very same qualities that often made them a target for bullies when they were adolescents in high school can often be assets in the workplace: single minded focus, intelligence, loyalty, dedication, a lot of knowledge about their topic of interest. These can all be turned into assets when they have a job where they need to know a lot about a particular topic and be able to focus for long periods of time on a particular task.

When they were younger, all they wanted to do was take apart toys and put them back together again. Fast forward ten years, and they have the makings to be a brilliant engineer.

Your Aspie teenager interested in the radio can become a DJ; your non-social techno-loving computer geek son can have a brilliant career in Silicon Valley doing computer work. Many Aspies have great computer and technical skills which can be very useful in those industries. Whatever interest an Aspie has, it can usually be translated into a career.

Most Aspies – by the term Aspie we mean a person with Asperger's Syndrome – have several qualities that can make them ideal employees. They are loyal; they usually have a great work ethic; they are often very concerned about being punctual and doing a good job, and they know a lot about the topic at hand, if it is something that is an interest of theirs. They will not be likely to spend all their time at work gossiping by the water cooler; instead, they will get things done.

These qualities can make a person with AS into an ideal employee; however, one has to find an employer that is willing to overlook the problems that an AS employee can present (not good at small talk or office politics, sensory issues, doesn't understand hidden rules) in order to see the gem they have and hire your AS kid in the first place. Or, they need to be coached in things like how to dress, how to make small talk, how to deal with office politics and so on in order to have a better chance of succeeding.

There is a rather high unemployment or underemployment (a term that refers to those who have jobs, but are too low paying or do not suit the person's capabilities) for adults with Asperger's. It is not uncommon for someone with a master's or higher degree to be un or underemployed. There are several problems that contribute to this issue and make the workplace a difficult place for a person with AS to be. Finding and keeping a job can be a difficult thing for a person with AS.

Specific Challenges for Young Adults with Asperger's in the Workplace

1. The interview

One of the biggest, if not *the* biggest, problems for adults with AS and employment is getting through the initial interview. Your kid with AS can be the brightest, sharpest person out there, can know the job inside out, but unless he can connect with the person doing the interview socially, and can come across well, they will never get past the front door.

People with AS do not do small talk well; might answer questions in a far too explicit manner or say nothing at all; give too much detail about their faults when it is not needed; not look people in the eye; and seem excessively nervous and fidgety, which is a sign to most interviewers that they are not prepared or right for the job – when, in fact, they are like that all the time.

People with AS can be trained in how to get through an interview, how to look people in the eye, how to answer questions the right way, but they are often going to have an air of anxiety pervading them that they can't get rid of no matter how much they try, and the interviewers pick up on this and often see them negatively for it. Not all, but a lot of them.

2. Office politics

As discussed earlier, people with AS do not do well reading hidden messages or understanding subtle social rules of a workplace. They might find themselves in some kind of pickle or social misunderstanding and have no idea how they got there. They might not do enough "schmoozing," or going to company Christmas parties and such, and be seen unfavorably for that, no matter how good their work is.

3. Finding a good fit

Finding something that suits interests and strengths. If the work is something the person with AS is not interested in, it will be hard for them to be motivated enough to focus on it. This is true for all people, of course, but can be particularly true for those with AS. On the flip side, if it is something they have an interest in, they will be extremely dedicated and loyal, and most likely far more productive than their fellow employees – they actually want to be there and enjoy the work.

4. Sensory issues

This can be one of the biggest problems for people with AS in the workplace. People talking in the next cubicle, even someone chewing gum or playing with a stapler, or swinging their foot back and forth – everything can be enormously distracting and bothersome to the adult with AS. Food and perfume smells can be hard to deal with. Bright lights, or not enough lights, uncomfortable chairs, computer screen glare, even the feel of the telephone as they are holding it – depending on their level of sensory integration difficulty, the workplace can be a very hostile and overwhelming environment indeed for the adult with AS. And, of course, jobs that demand too much social interaction from an adult with AS can be draining and almost impossible for them to deal with.

As mentioned before, asking for a separate office or trying to work from home as much as possible can solve some of these issues.

5. Organization, understanding instruction

As mentioned before, some adults with AS find it hard to organize and understand information unless presented in a very logical and explicit way. Information and instructions have to be presented very clearly and often written down step by step. No assumptions can be made. An adult with AS will often be overwhelmed with an instruction to "get to work," look around them, see everyone working, and have no idea what they are supposed to be doing (and be too scared to ask), if information has not been presented clearly.

Careers that are Best Suited for People with Asperger's

As mentioned before, adults with AS do have certain traits that lend themselves particularly well to certain fields.

Some of the things one should look for when looking for a job for someone with AS are the following:

- They are able to work as independently as possible (not a lot of team meetings or working with others)

- A career that requires attention to detail, patterns, or doing the same thing over and over (not right for all with AS , but fits many)

Best jobs for people with Aspergers

- Computer programming
- Math
- Statistics
- Writing
- Languages
- Research
- working in a library as a reference librarian
- Professor at a college
- Engineering
- The arts if they are into this

Worst jobs:

- Anything that requires constant interaction with people

- Requires working under too much pressure, having to work too fast or multi-task

As an example, a cashier would likely be a bad choice. A cashier has to interact with and perform a large number of things all at once while being friendly and communicating at the same time. This requires speed, multi-tasking, and too much social interaction – NOT strengths of a person with AS.

Some young adults with Asperger's are able to work, and many are not. Some have too many sensory issues to be able to focus in a busy, noisy workplace for eight hours a day. Some can work part time, but not full time. Some do better if they can find a job working from home, or working outdoors; being a park ranger, painting someone's house, landscaping, even being a lifeguard can be easier than trying to focus in an office environment.

Some people with Asperger's have a lot of trouble understanding the social rules and therefore will have trouble getting and keeping jobs. But others manage to flourish in the workplace; they have jobs where the rules of conduct are clear; not a lot of social interaction is required, or if it is, it is done with understanding and helpful people and with breaks in between. A young adult with Asperger's can indeed succeed in the workplace especially if they are working in an area of special interest to them and have lots of support and coaching in areas where they lack knowledge or skills.

8. The College Issue

Should My Child Go to College? Where?

Working is an important part of a young adult's post-high school life, but so is college. One of the first decisions that often has to be made when planning for a teen with Asperger's post high school life is, should they go to college? And if so, should they live at home or go away to school?

Your guidance counselor and teachers that know your teen well will be able to best help you with this decision – and of course what your teen wants should be factored in as well.

Some of the skills that a teen will need in order to live on their own at college are:

- Self-care skills – like showering, dressing

- Cooking skill – knowing how to cook basic foods or at least remembering to eat

- Basic communication skills – so they can figure out how to get their needs met and form new relationships at their school

- Anxiety management skills – do they know how to manage their anxiety more or less okay?

- Handling meltdowns – can they recover from meltdowns on their own? Do they have many meltdowns? How often do they get very upset when things don't go their way, and can they recover from these upsets?

  If your child is having many meltdowns on a regular basis, going away to school probably isn't feasible; all the changes and responsibilities of being in a new place and having to live with other people will probably throw them too much. If they have some anxiety, but have coping skills to be able to recover from it (cognitive restructuring, engaging in calming activities, seeking help from a support person), then likely they will be able to manage living on their own.

Other issues with living at college include:

- Living in a single room or to have roommates?

- What supports will they need in the classroom?

- How big of a college? Smaller colleges tend to work better as there is a more supportive, friendly atmosphere, and professors tend to know their students personally, instead of them being just a number.

Often there are a variety of living options on campus, from singles to doubles to apartments; and usually, there are disability offices that can offer a wide variety of academic supports. Some academic supports include extra time on tests, private tutoring, the ability to take tests in separate rooms if a quieter environment or extra support is needed, note takers, and so on.

If you feel your teen is not able to live on their own at college, you might want to consider a community college. This way, your teen can still live at home and get support from you at home, but go to classes and earn a degree just the same. Most community colleges will also have disability offices that offer accommodations such as listed above.

Six Issues to Consider When Choosing a College

1. Size

Is a 30,000 person university going to be too overwhelming for your child? Would a small liberal arts college be a more nurturing environment? Or would the size and added resources of a bigger school be good for your teen?

2. Interest

What does your teen want to study? What schools have programs in this? What are some possible back up ideas to study if the preferred one doesn't work out?

3. Distance

How far is your teen comfortable being from your house? How far are you comfortable having them away? How would they get home on holidays (driving, you pick them up, plane, train?)

4. Student body

It is important to consider the student body of any college you are looking at. Is it mostly liberal in values, or more conservative? Does it have a reputation for elitism and snobbery, or does it seem to have an open minded and tolerant student body? How much activism is there? What do students do in their free time? What are the extracurricular clubs and opportunities like? All of these should be matched to your teen's interests as closely as possible. Schools with reputations for diversity or open mindedness will probably be more accepting of your teen's differences than schools with reputations for cutthroat academic performance, elitism or highly competitive atmospheres.

5. Climate and location

Does your teen want to be in a northern climate, or is the south okay? How does he do in very hot (or cold) weather? What is the town the school is located in like? Do you need a car to get places, or can you walk? Are there grocery stores nearby, and things to do? Does the town feel safe to you?

6. Disability services

Depending on how extensive your teen's support needs are, you may want to choose a college with a good reputation for providing disability services. You can usually talk to the disability service offices in colleges to get a feel for what they offer and how extensive, or not, their experience working with students with Asperger's is. Some colleges might already have support groups for students with Asperger's if they have enough of them.

This website lists several colleges who responded to a survey about how autism and Asperger's-friendly their colleges or universities were, and may be helpful in learning what accommodations are available for those with Asperger's:

http://www.larsperner.com/autism/colleges.htm

How to Prepare for College: Tips from a College Instructor on the Autism Spectrum

We can usually learn a lot from those who have already lived a particular situation; in this case, a woman named Maureen Johnson is a college instructor in Illinois, and also

someone who has Asperger's. She provides many insights into how to prepare for and succeed in college for those with Asperger's. Some of her tips, courtesy of the Autism About.com website include the following:
[http://autism.about.com/od/transitioncollegejobs/a/mjohnsontips.htm]

"1. Obtain certification of your ASD from your medical professional. In order to obtain accommodations on a college campus (such as disability support services), you will probably be required to have documentation of your ASD from a physician, neurologist, or psychiatrist.

2. If you are planning on living in a dorm, you may want to let the administration know about your ASD or request a private room. If you are someone who is extremely sensitive to external stimuli (light, sound, etc), you may want to be placed in a "study floor" instead of a "sorority wing." Or, if possible, you may want to request a private room so that you have a little more control over your environment.

3. Let your professors know of your ASD and what may be helpful to you. If possible, arrange a meeting with your professors before the beginning of the semester, but no later than the first week. They will probably respect your honesty and the initiative you are taking in your courses. Also, don't hesitate to ask for help. As an instructor, I am always willing to help someone who asks for it.

4. Without delay, locate the disability support services on campus. This is very important, as they will likely be the professionals who will arrange (or provide verification) for you to receive necessary accommodations to perform well in your courses.

5. Join an activity to meet people with similar interests to your own. Socializing is not something that always comes easily to people with an ASD. Think of those

activities you enjoy or in which you have succeeded. There are bound to be groups or clubs focusing on that activity.

6. Consider taking a few classes online. Students with an ASD may be overwhelmed by the harsh lighting and noise from a classroom. You may want to check and see if a couple of your required classes may be taken online. However, be advised that taking classes online actually requires more self-discipline than in a traditional classroom."

Challenges You May Face

What are the biggest challenges teens with Asperger's face when they go to college?

We've talked a lot about how to choose a college and tips on how to deal with particular issues that could arise for a teen with Asperger's who goes to college. But let's talk more specifically about the biggest potential challenges that students with Asperger's face when they go to college. The more you are aware of the potential problems, the more tools you will have to be able to solve them when they come up.

1. Social issues

By far, the biggest issues that teens with Asperger's face when they go to college is figuring out how to navigate the social environment. Doing the academic work may be easy, but figuring out how to say hi to someone in the hallways, how to start conversations with peers, and how to solve conflicts that arise in the dorms can be very difficult. Aspie teens are often not good at breaking into group conversations, starting new conversations, keeping conversations going, etc. They may find it difficult to make friends and end up feeling isolated. Special interest groups and counseling can help with this.

2. Distance

If your teen has traveled a long way from home to go to his or her college, feelings of loneliness and of being out of place are common. They don't know, at first, where anything is; everything seems very unfamiliar. Visits home can help at first; phone calls can help a lot; and of course, time will do the most to heal this particular problem.

3. Sensory overload

Colleges can be very overwhelming from a sensory perspective. There are hundreds or even thousands of people walking around, talking, laughing, doing their thing around you at every minute. There is lots of noise, commotion, smells, activity. It can be overwhelming at times. Classrooms can be loud; hallways can be loud. It can be hard to concentrate in class, or when taking tests, due to noise. It can be hard to sleep in the dorms or study due to noise. Students with AS can ask for special quiet rooms to take tests in, and try to seek out quieter areas of campus such as the library to spend most of their time in if they have trouble with noise levels or other sensory concerns.

4. Academic concerns

Some teens with AS may need private tutoring or other accommodations to help them keep up with their classes, or personal coaches or counselors to help them stay organized enough to turn in all their work and complete all the necessary daily activities.

Final College Remarks

Well, there you have it: the good, the bad and the ugly about college for people on the autism spectrum. College is not for everyone. There are many benefits to a college experience; besides being a useful entry into the work world, it can provide invaluable social experience and build an AS student's self-esteem considerably. But the downside is it can be a very stressful environment for some people, and not tolerable for some. Only you and your teen can decide if college is a good option for your teen with Asperger's.

9. What if My Teen Can Neither Work nor Attend College?

For some people, neither working or college is an option for them. Their sensory issues may be too great; their anxiety problems too huge; their adjustment problems too significant. Or they may simply not be able to work and not interested in college.

Some might do volunteer work instead. Some might have to go on disability to get by, and fill their time with their interests, with support groups, therapy, or as much socialization as they can get. (Or some might not be interested in anything social at all.) Some might spend their time on various hobbies of various intensity; some might need support workers, some might not. Most will find some degree of happiness in their life, most likely from their special interests or hobbies, whether they are able to work or not. Everyone has different degrees of what society would call "success," but there are at least some social service nets to catch those people who cannot manage to work on their own, and they can usually manage to develop a somewhat satisfying life working around their problems and focusing on their interests in these cases.

Sheltered Workshops

There are options for those with Asperger's who are not able to work. One option that exists is called a sheltered workshop. These are usually organizations that have jobs that people with disabilities can do that offer a lot of support. One organization defines sheltered workshops this way: "Sheltered workshops are state supported vocational programs designed to provide work for persons with mental retardation/developmental disabilities."
[http://www.rcomo.org/whatisasw.htm]

They go on to describe the value of sheltered workshops further:

- "Pay Check" allows the handicapped to perform a service for society by earning a portion of their livelihood.

- "Responsibility" gives them the responsibility of coming to work and doing a job.

- "Asset to Business" performs a service to competitive industry in jobs that are labor intensive.

- "Socialization" working side by side with their buddies.

In addition it's probably the greatest Respite program ever designed for parents and guardians, because they have the peace of mind that their son or daughter is safe, secure and a productive member of society."
[http://www.rcomo.org/whatisasw.htm]

Sheltered workshops can be found in most cities. Ask your local Autism Society of America chapter, or your doctor, for referrals to local places.

Other forms of supported employment are also available; oftentimes those with disabilities such as Asperger's qualify for a job coach who can be there while they work a job to ask any questions or to give any support necessary.

Living Arrangements for Adults with Asperger's

Some adults with autism can live on their own successfully in their own apartments. Others need different degrees of help. Here are some of the options:

Supported Living: These are situations where the person with Asperger's lives mostly independently in an apartment, but has access to a support person if he needs it. He can call that person, or maybe there's a live in person, whenever a problem arises that he can't solve himself. Or perhaps there is someone who visits a few times a week. Perhaps there are many people with disabilities living in the same building and a support person or two available to all of them. It's living on your own, just with a little support. Often people in supported living can go to work and engage in various daily activities, but just with a little help on the side.

Group Homes This is when several people with disabilities, including autism or Asperger's, all live in the same house, usually an average of around five or six, and have live in staff people who take care of them and help them with daily living activities, such as cooking and cleaning. The quality, structure, and strictness of such places varies greatly; you will need to research a group home very thoroughly before deciding on one. Some group homes have very strict rules and do not afford their residents very much independence; others are looser. Some are better than others at teaching necessary life skills to their residents. There have been many reports of abuse at group homes, but this is not something that happens in all of them; again, you just need to get a lot of references, talk to parents who have kids in it, and observe for yourself as best as you can to make sure it is a good fit with your child.

Peer Mentoring Some parents are getting an apartment or house for their child, and then hiring a peer to live there with their child. In exchange for living there rent free, the peer helps the person with autism with minor problems that might come up, such as with bills or other household problems; but the person with autism lives independently. Some states have programs where they pay people to live with a disabled person for just that purpose.

Other Residential Options include different kinds of facilities where the needs of the person with autism can be attended to, depending on the level of severity of these needs. There are residential schools with dorms that accept more severely affected autistic kids at age 18, give them programming to teach them life skills and social skills, try to give them a sense of community, and fulfill all their other basic living needs. Sometimes the person goes home on the weekends to see their family, sometimes they don't. And, of course, there are still mental hospitals or institutions where the most severely affected and hard to manage autistic people may end up; but few parents want their child in such a setting, and that is usually a last resort.

Living at Home is also an option for many adults with Asperger's. Home is familiar to people with Asperger's and some parents don't mind continuing to care for their child as he gets older. A lot of people with autism spectrum disorders can still work outside the home if they get the support they need while living at home. If a person is receiving disability benefits from the government, this can make the financing part of this situation easier on the parents. Many parents feel like they can take the best care of their child even into adulthood and feel this is the best option for their child. Other options might not be practical depending on the situation of the particular person.

What services are available to adults with Asperger's?

Do not fear, there is still some help your young Asperger's adult can get when he reaches adult age. The following are various things that can help adults with Asperger's.

Social security benefits: Many people with autism spectrum disorders are eligible for disability benefits; a certain amount of money that is paid to them every month. This usually differs per person and situation. Some people get SSI, Supplemental Security Income, which is a smaller amount of money used to offset living expenses. Others can get SSDI, Social Security Disability Income, which is usually a larger amount. Generally, the more you have worked, the more you are eligible to get. This can be a necessary supplement for a person with autism who has difficulty securing and maintaining employment to have; it can provide at least some vestiges of an independent life.

Health insurance: If your child receives disability benefits, usually health insurance in the form of Medicare is eventually included in this; Medicare will help pay for doctor's visits and medications. Your child may also be eligible for Medicaid, another federal program to help people who are low income or disabled to have health insurance.

Section 8: Not just for people with disabilities, this is a program intended to help with the costs of renting an apartment for people who would not be able to afford it any other way.

People in this program usually pay about 30% of their income once they are accepted. There are usually very long waiting lists to get into this program, usually even up to a year or two, so it's best to put your name on the waiting list early. It can be confusing as sometimes there are only certain times a year that a Section 8 office will accept new names to a waiting list, but it is a worthwhile thing to try.

Another thing to look into is apartment buildings that have their own subsidies attached. These are apartments where, if you qualify, you will only have to pay a certain percentage of your income to live there. The waiting lists are not usually as long as Section 8, but depending on where you apply, it is not always easy to get one of those. If you can get one, though, it can be a really good thing.

In home support services: There are many agencies that provide in home support services for a variety of needs, including those of adults with autism. This can be a useful thing to someone trying to live independently but who needs a little more help.

Support groups: Adults with autism spectrum disorders may benefit from attending support groups. Some are run by therapists and you have to pay for; others are run by lay people or other autistic people, and are free. Some focus on teaching social skills; others focus on conversation and giving autistic adults a place to have a social gathering and meet other people. Meeting other autistic adults can be a great boon to one's morale. Search the Internet to find support groups near where you live. Three great sites for this include:

www.meetup.com

www.asperger.org/Prof_and_Parent_Support.asp

www.yellowpagesforkids.com

Final Remarks

In closing, being a teenager can be an exciting, although challenging, time. When your teen gets to be 16 or 17, it is time to start planning for their future. Some teens with Asperger's skip college and go straight to work; some op to go to a community college; many will decide to go away to college like their peers. Some are not able to either work or go to college. It all depends on your child's unique strengths and weaknesses; a large number of factors should be taken into consideration while making a plan for their future. After years of trying to plan for every contingency and make plans for their education, you are now tasked with having to plan their future; but with the years of experience you have already had in taking care of your child's needs, don't worry, you will do just fine. Your Aspie teen will be able to find their place in the world in time.

Bonus Report: How to Get Into the College of Your Choice

So you've decided your teen is college material, and you even have an idea of where he or she should go. Great, but have you considered the following things to prepare your teen with Asperger's for college?

1. Standardized tests

SATs and other standardized test used as an entrance criteria for many colleges. Most students take them in the junior year of high school. They can be retaken if necessary. They contains verbal and math sections. Some standardized tests are subject tests and/or have writing sections. Some parents pay for prep courses to get their kids ready for these standardized tests. Depending on how your teen with Asperger's usually does with tests, this may be a very good idea.

Some people don't take tests well; some have enormous testing anxiety. A benefit of a test prep course is that it often lowers the anxiety level by allowing a student to understand what the test entails. You can get practice tests to do with your teen to get them used to the test and format. I recommend this because you want to try to ease their anxiety about taking the test. Make sure your teen has a proper breakfast before the test, and that he or she gets enough sleep the night before.

If your teen does poorly on standardized tests, there are some colleges that no longer consider the SAT in their application process. Definitely consider these colleges if your son or daughter does poorly on standardized tests.

2. Grades

Are your teen's grades good enough to get into the college he or she desires? Many parents want their children to go to the most prestigious or competitive colleges. But for an AS student this may not be the best idea. Ideally, you do not want your child to struggle or fall behind. AS students have so many more issues to deal with that typical students do – sensory issues, dealing with change, social problems – just to name a few.

Most colleges will tell you the average grades of their entering freshman. I recommend that your child fall in the upper 33% of the entering freshman class as far as high school grades are concerned. If the cut off for the top 33% is a 3.8 grade point average, and your child has a 3.2 grade point average, realize that they will be up against stiff competition and may struggle to maintain good grades in college. When they graduate, an employer is likely to look at your child's grades because their work history will be limited. It is better to have an "A" or "B" average from a less well known school than to be a "C" or "D" student from a more competitive college.

3. Letters of recommendation

As your teen goes through high school, remember that they will eventually need a letter of recommendation (or several) from teachers for their college application. Try to get a few teachers who really know your teen well and who can speak to their unique strengths and abilities to write a letter of recommendation. A personal, well thought out letter will count for a lot more than the form letters that some teachers use.

Bonus Report: 7 Secrets to Succeed in College with Asperger's Syndrome

Once you've chosen the college and signed up for the classes, now the hard work begins – figuring out how to get along in college while dealing with social gaffes, sensory issues and being just plain overwhelmed. College can be hard for even typical students at first, but for those with Asperger's, there are several additional challenges and curveballs to contend with. Here are some tips that an AS student will likely find very beneficial for succeeding in college.

1. Make connections with professors

It is very important to make connections with whomever you can. These will become your lifeline. Try to befriend your professors   they are often much easier to interact with than your peers. Typically, this is easier in a small college, so I recommend choosing a college small enough where you will be able to have a relationship with your professors.

Stay after class and talk to them about the assignment or a particular idea you had about one of the topics from class. Comment about the weather. Ask their opinion of school wide issues. Any kind of repeated small talk leads to a feeling of connection, and a genuine friendship. When you need to talk about more serious issues or need help with something, you will have natural allies.

These connections will keep you from feeling too lonely, and give you a sense of connection to and belonging within the college. You will most likely find doing this with professors much easier than with your peers. A personal connections with professors is also very important in landing your first job. A great letter of recommendation from a professor can have a lot of influence over a potential employer. AS graduates often have problems in job interviews. A sympathetic professor who got to know you personally can help explain your differences and strengths in a letter to a potential employer – and most professors are very happy to write these letters for students, especially if you were really passionate about the material you were taught.

2. Accept that you are different

The second most important thing I can bestow on you in order to be able to succeed in college is to accept that you are different. Don't waste all your time comparing yourself to others. Know that you may appear different, talk different, walk different, have different interests, yada yada. It's not worth beating yourself up over it. You've known this for a long time, it's old news. If you choose the right college, the student body won't care that you're different. Look for smaller, quirky colleges with a more welcoming student body.

> As one AS student told me, *"At my college, I was quite self conscious my first couple of years, but eventually grew into myself and didn't care that I appeared different. Instead, I reveled in it. This gave me more confidence when interacting with my peers and helped me to make friends."*

3. Follow your passions

Take classes in what you are truly interested in, not what other people tell you to. Boredom is the most surefire way to fail academically. Follow your passions. Make the material your own. When you are assigned a project or a paper, think to yourself, "What do I want to say about the world, or myself? What do I want to find out about the world or myself? How I can express this in this paper in a meaningful way?" Find something that engages you, and you will excel academically and really get something out of the process in the meantime. One AS student said,

> *"At my college, I really enjoyed when we got to do portfolios in my psychology classes. We were allowed to express our learning of the material in any way we wished: through essays, song lyrics, paintings, research papers, or whatever we liked. I was able to really explore myself and the world around me while doing these portfolios."*

4. Anticipate and overcome sensory problems

College can be a sensory nightmare, but only if you let it. You must learn to work around sensory concerns. If noise is a problem while you are taking tests, ask to take tests in a separate room or the learning center. If you have a problem with perfumes, have the teacher ask the class not to wear any. If you tend to get overwhelmed while being out and about on a busy college campus, get a Walkman to listen to while you walk around. This will soothe you and give you something to concentrate on.

Figure out the way you relax best and work time into your schedule to do it. Find a nice, quiet place on campus that you can retreat to when you need to.

> *"For me, that was the basement of my school library. I personally had trouble going to sleep at*

135

night when I could hear any noise at all coming from any of the other dorm rooms. So I scheduled late classes and made a point to stay up until two or three in the morning when I was sure everyone else had gone to sleep. Unorthodox, yes, but it worked throughout the time I was at my college."

5. Find enjoyment

Find something you enjoy, and do it regularly. Make sure you leave time to relax. Don't stress out if you don't have anyone to do it with. There is no law stating you can't go out to dinner by yourself or to a movie alone. Sometimes, it is even more enjoyable that way. Take yourself out on the town.

"I used smoothies as rewards for difficult tasks, and regularly went into town by myself. I wandered around and forgot about school for a while."

6. Get organized!

Organization. Knowing yourself and your patterns, and **having a routine**, is key to succeeding. What time of day do you work best? Morning or night, before dinner or after? Do you work best under the pressure of deadlines or do you need to break tasks into smaller, more manageable chunks? Do you need an area with no distractions to work in, or does some amount of activity stimulate your thinking process? These are all important things to know about yourself. Have a schedule of when you will do all your work, and stick to it. Invest in binders and keep work neatly labeled where you can find it. Try to work around the same time every day.

7. Ask for help

Finally, and this is very important, ask for help if you need it. Most colleges have learning centers where you can get extra tutoring or other accommodations. Don't be afraid to be a pest when asking teachers to clarify assignments – it's better than getting a bad grade. Utilize email to ask questions of professors if talking to face to face is too difficult. **Make sure you have a source of support.** The counseling center in your school can be very useful to help you deal with the myriad stresses of a college career. Make sure you have someone to talk to, whether that person be a friend, a professor, family member, or whoever.

If you follow all of those tips, I think that you will find you will really enjoy your college experience. Your college years are particularly notable because not only are you learning a ton of stuff academically, but you are also growing so much as a person. You're learning how to live on your own, how to interact with others, how to discipline yourself and stay motivated. You're learning about things you are interested in, and new ways to express yourself. You're building an identity for yourself. I wish you all the luck as you travel down this important path!

Bonus Report: Step-by-Step Survey to Measure the Bullying Problem in Your School

Many schools will turn a blind eye towards bullying. They simply do not want to acknowledge the severity of the problem. Or they may think that bullying is a rare and isolated event. Many students know otherwise. They understand that bullying is rampant in many schools. They are tormented, day after day by bullies – and the school does nothing about it.

Other times, after a parent or group of parents complains about the bullying problem in their school, the administration does *something*, but the problem does not go away.

In both of these cases, it is much easier to gain the attention of the school administrators and the board of education if you are armed with data. It is impossible to claim that bullying is an isolated problem if survey data proves otherwise. Below, we show an example survey that you can easily type up, photocopy and distribute to students. You will need the help of your school's administration in most cases. But if they refuse to help, ask your son or daughter's teachers if they will pass out the survey to the students they teach. At least you will have *some* data to prove your point.

Once you have data that shows how much of a problem bullying is in your school, it is much more difficult for administrators to ignore the problem.

Here is a survey which you could use. Please feel free to modify it to your specific situation. Adapted from a survey by The National Crime Prevention Council.

Bullying Survey

DIRECTIONS: Please mark the best answers to the following questions. You may have more than one best answer for some questions. You do not have to put your name on the paper.

Name (optional)_____

1. Have you ever been bullied?
    ☐ Yes
    ☐ No

If you answered yes, how often did someone bully you?
    ☐ Occasionally
    ☐ Often
    ☐ Every day

Where did it happen?

    ☐ School
    ☐ Park
    ☐ Home
    ☐ Neighborhood
    ☐ Somewhere else

If it happened at school, where?

    ☐ Hallway
    ☐ Classroom
    ☐ Playground
    ☐ Cafeteria
    ☐ Bathroom
    ☐ Somewhere else

2. Have you seen other students being bullied at school?

- ☐ Yes
- ☐ No

If you answered yes, how often did it happen?

- ☐ Occasionally
- ☐ Often
- ☐ Every day

Where have you seen other students bullied?

- ☐ Hallway
- ☐ Classroom
- ☐ Playground
- ☐ Cafeteria
- ☐ Bathroom
- ☐ Somewhere else

3. What kinds of things have bullies done to you or to someone you know?

- ☐ Called names
- ☐ Threatened
- ☐ Stole or damaged something
- ☐ Shoved, kicked, or hit
- ☐ Ignored

4. How much of a problem is bullying for you?

- ☐ Very much
- ☐ Not much
- ☐ None

5. On the back of this paper, list some of the actions you think parents, teachers, and other adults could perform to stop bullying.

Bonus Report: A Guide to the Individualized Education Program

Office of Special Education and Rehabilitative Services

U.S. Department of Education

Credits

This guide was developed by the U.S. Department of Education, with the assistance of the National Information Center for Children and Youth with Disabilities (NICHCY). The Department staff contributing to this guide include: Debra Price-Ellingstad, JoLeta Reynolds, Larry Ringer, Ruth Ryder, and Suzanne Sheridan, under the direction of Judith E. Heumann, Kenneth Warlick, and Curtis Richards.

Editor: Lisa Küpper, NICHCY

Production: Jean Kohanek, NICHCY

Disability Art: Madison, Moore, disabilityart.com

Additional copies of this guide are available from:

ED Pubs
Editorial Publications Center
U.S. Department of Education
P.O. Box 1398
Jessup, MD 20794-1398
(877) 4-ED-PUBS
(877) 576-7734 TTY
(301) 470-1244 Fax
http://www.ed.gov/pubs/edpubs.html

To obtain this publication in an alternate format (braille, large print, audio cassette, or disk), please contact Katie Mincey, Director of the Alternate Format Center, at (202) 260-9895, or via e-mail at Katie_Mincey@ed.gov.
This document is also available online at:
http://www.ed.gov/offices/OSERS

Contents

The federal regulations for Individualized Education Programs and additional guidance on the content of the IEP.

Introduction

Each public school child who receives special education and related services must have an Individualized Education Program (IEP). Each IEP must be designed for one student and must be a truly *individualized* document. The IEP creates an opportunity for teachers, parents, school administrators, related services personnel, and students (when appropriate) to work together to improve educational results for children with disabilities. The IEP is the cornerstone of a quality education for each child with a disability.

To create an effective IEP, parents, teachers, other school staff--and often the student--must come together to look closely at the student's unique needs. These individuals pool knowledge, experience, and commitment to design an educational program that will help the student be involved in, and progress in, the general curriculum. The IEP guides the delivery of special education supports and services for the student with a disability. Without a doubt, writing--and implementing--an effective IEP requires teamwork.

This guide explains the IEP process, which we consider to be one of the most critical elements to ensure effective teaching, learning, and better results for all children with disabilities. The guide is designed to help teachers, parents, and others--in fact, anyone involved in the education of a child with a disability--develop and carry out an IEP. The information in this guide is based on what is required by our nation's special education law--the Individuals with Disabilities Education Act, or IDEA.

The IDEA requires certain information to be included in each child's IEP. It is useful to know, however, that states and local school systems often include additional information in IEPs in order to document that they have met certain aspects of federal or state law. The flexibility that states and school systems have to design their own IEP forms is one reason why IEP forms may look different from school system to school system or state to state. Yet each IEP is critical in the education of a child with a disability.

The Basic Special Education Process Under IDEA

The writing of each student's IEP takes place within the larger picture of the special education process under IDEA. Before taking a detailed look at the IEP, it may be helpful to look briefly at how a student is identified as having a disability and needing special education and related services and, thus, an IEP.

Step 1. Child is identified as possibly needing special education and related services.

"Child Find." The state must identify, locate, and evaluate all children with disabilities in the state who need special education and related services. To do so, states conduct "Child Find" activities. A child may be identified by "Child Find," and parents may be asked if the "Child Find" system can evaluate their child. Parents can also call the "Child Find" system and ask that their child be evaluated. Or--

Referral or request for evaluation. A school professional may ask that a child be evaluated to see if he or she has a disability. Parents may also contact the child's teacher or other school professional to ask that their child be evaluated. This request may be verbal or in writing. Parental consent is needed before the child may be evaluated. Evaluation needs to be completed within a reasonable time after the parent gives consent.

Step 2. Child is evaluated.

The evaluation must assess the child in all areas related to the child's suspected disability. The evaluation results will be used to decide the child's eligibility for special education and related services and to make decisions about an appropriate educational program for the child. If the

147

parents disagree with the evaluation, they have the right to take their child for an Independent Educational Evaluation (IEE). They can ask that the school system pay for this IEE.

Step 3. Eligibility is decided.

A group of qualified professionals and the parents look at the child's evaluation results. Together, they decide if the child is a "child with a disability," as defined by IDEA. Parents may ask for a hearing to challenge the eligibility decision.

Step 4. Child is found eligible for services.

If the child is found to be a "child with a disability," as defined by IDEA, he or she is eligible for special education and related services. Within 30 calendar days after a child is determined eligible, the IEP team must meet to write an IEP for the child.

Once the student has been found eligible for services, the IEP must be written. The two steps below *summarize* what is involved in writing the IEP.   This guide will look at these two steps in much greater detail in the following section.

Step 5. IEP meeting is scheduled.

The school system schedules and conducts the IEP meeting. School staff must:

- contact the participants, including the parents;
- notify parents early enough to make sure they have an opportunity to attend;
- schedule the meeting at a time and place agreeable to parents and the school;
- tell the parents the purpose, time, and location of the meeting;
- tell the parents who will be attending; and

- tell the parents that they may invite people to the meeting who have knowledge or special expertise about the child.

Step 6. IEP meeting is held and the IEP is written.

The IEP team gathers to talk about the child's needs and write the student's IEP. Parents and the student (when appropriate) are part of the team. If the child's placement is decided by a different group, the parents must be part of that group as well.

Before the school system may provide special education and related services to the child for the first time, the parents must give consent. The child begins to receive services as soon as possible after the meeting.

If the parents do not agree with the IEP and placement, they may discuss their concerns with other members of the IEP team and try to work out an agreement. If they still disagree, parents can ask for mediation, or the school may offer mediation. Parents may file a complaint with the state education agency and may request a due process hearing, at which time mediation must be available.

Here is a brief summary of what happens after the IEP is written.

Step 7. Services are provided.

The school makes sure that the child's IEP is being carried out as it was written. Parents are given a copy of the IEP. Each of the child's teachers and service providers has access to the IEP and knows his or her specific responsibilities for carrying out the IEP. This includes the accommodations, modifications, and supports that must be provided to the child, in keeping with the IEP.

Step 8. Progress is measured and reported to parents.

The child's progress toward the annual goals is measured, as stated in the IEP. His or her parents are regularly informed of their child's progress and whether that progress is enough for the child to achieve the goals by the end of the year. These progress reports must be given to parents at least as often as parents are informed of their nondisabled children's progress.

Step 9. IEP is reviewed.

The child's IEP is reviewed by the IEP team at least once a year, or more often if the parents or school ask for a review. If necessary, the IEP is revised. Parents, as team members, must be invited to attend these meetings. Parents can make suggestions for changes, can agree or disagree with the IEP goals, and agree or disagree with the placement.

If parents do not agree with the IEP and placement, they may discuss their concerns with other members of the IEP team and try to work out an agreement. There are several options, including additional testing, an independent evaluation, or asking for mediation (if available) or a due process hearing. They may also file a complaint with the state education agency.

Step 10. Child is reevaluated.

At least every three years the child must be reevaluated. This evaluation is often called a "triennial." Its purpose is to find out if the child continues to be a "child with a disability," as defined by IDEA, and what the child's educational needs are. However, the child must be reevaluated more often if conditions warrant or if the child's parent or teacher asks for a reevaluation.

A Closer Look at the IEP

Clearly, the IEP is a very important document for children with disabilities and for those who are involved in educating them. Done correctly, the IEP should improve teaching, learning, and results. Each child's IEP describes, among other things, the educational program that has been designed to meet that child's unique needs. This part of the guide looks closely at how the IEP is written and by whom, and what information it must, at a minimum, contain.

Contents of the IEP

By law, the IEP must include certain information about the child and the educational program designed to meet his or her unique needs. In a nutshell, this information is:

- ■ *Current performance.* The IEP must state how the child is currently doing in school (known as *present levels of educational performance*). This information usually comes from the evaluation results such as classroom tests and assignments, individual tests given to decide eligibility for services or during reevaluation, and observations made by parents, teachers, related service providers, and other school staff. The statement about "current performance" includes how the child's disability affects his or her involvement and progress in the general curriculum.
- ■ *Annual goals.* These are goals that the child can reasonably accomplish in a year. The goals are broken down into short-term *objectives or benchmarks*. Goals may be academic, address social or behavioral needs, relate to physical needs, or address other educational needs. The goals must be measurable-meaning that it must be possible to measure whether the student has achieved the goals.
- ■ *Special education and related services.* The IEP must list the special education and related services to be provided to the child or on behalf of the child. This

151

includes supplementary aids and services that the child needs. It also includes modifications (changes) to the program or supports for school personnel-such as training or professional development-that will be provided to assist the child.

- **Participation with nondisabled children.** The IEP must explain the extent (if any) to which the child will *not* participate with nondisabled children in the regular class and other school activities.

- **Participation in state and district-wide tests.** Most states and districts give achievement tests to children in certain grades or age groups. The IEP must state what modifications in the administration of these tests the child will need. If a test is not appropriate for the child, the IEP must state why the test is not appropriate and how the child will be tested instead.

- **Dates and places.** The IEP must state when services will begin, how often they will be provided, where they will be provided, and how long they will last.

- **Transition service needs.** Beginning when the child is age 14 (or younger, if appropriate), the IEP must address (within the applicable parts of the IEP) the courses he or she needs to take to reach his or her post-school goals. A statement of transition services needs must also be included in each of the child's subsequent IEPs.

- **Needed transition services.** Beginning when the child is age 16 (or younger, if appropriate), the IEP must state what transition services are needed to help the child prepare for leaving school.

- **Age of majority.** Beginning at least one year before the child reaches the age of majority, the IEP must include a statement that the student has been told of any rights that will transfer to him or her at the age of majority. (This statement would be needed only in states that transfer rights at the age of majority.)

- **Measuring progress.** The IEP must state how the child's progress will be measured and how parents will be informed of that progress.

152

More information will be given about these IEP parts later in this guide. A sample IEP form will be presented, along with the federal regulations describing the "Content of the IEP," to help you gain a fuller understanding of what type of information is important to capture about a child in an IEP. It is useful to understand that each child's IEP is different. The document is prepared for *that child only*. It describes the *individualized* education program designed to meet *that* child's needs.

Additional State and School-System Content

States and school systems have a great deal of flexibility about the information they require in an IEP. Some states and school systems have chosen to include in the IEP additional information to document their compliance with other state and federal requirements. (Federal law requires that school districts maintain documentation to demonstrate their compliance with federal requirements.) Generally speaking, extra elements in IEPs may be included to document that the state or school district has met certain aspects of federal or state law, such as:

- holding the meeting to write, review, and, if necessary, revise a child's IEP in a timely manner;
- providing parents with a copy of the procedural safeguards they have under the law;
- placing the child in the least restrictive environment; and
- obtaining the parents' consent.

IEP Forms in Different Places

While the law tells us what information must be included in the IEP, it does *not* specify what the IEP should look like. No one form or approach or appearance is required or even suggested. Each state may decide what its IEPs will look like. In some states individual school systems design their own IEP forms.

Thus, across the United States, many different IEP forms are used. What is important is that each form be as clear and as useful as possible, so that parents, educators, related service providers, administrators, and others can easily *use* the form to write and implement effective IEPs for their students with disabilities.

The IEP Team Members

By law, certain individuals must be involved in writing a child's Individualized Education Program. These are:

- the child's parents;
- at least one of the child's special education teachers or providers;
- at least one of the child's regular education teachers (if the student is, or may be, participating in the regular education environment);
- a representative of the school system;
- an individual who can interpret the evaluation results;
- representatives of any other agencies that may be responsible for paying for or providing transition services (if the student is 16 years or, if appropriate, younger);
- the student, as appropriate, and
- other individuals who have knowledge or special expertise about the child.

Note that an IEP team member may fill more than one of the team positions if properly qualified and designated. For example, the school system representative may also be the person who can interpret the child's evaluation results.

These people must work together as a team to write the child's IEP. A meeting to write the IEP must be held within 30 calendar days of deciding that the child is eligible for special education and related services.

Each team member brings important information to the IEP meeting. Members share their information and work together to write the child's Individualized Education Program. Each person's information adds to the team's understanding of the child and what services the child needs.

Parents are key members of the IEP team. They know their child very well and can talk about their child's strengths and needs as well as their ideas for enhancing their child's education. They can offer insight into how their child learns, what his or her interests are, and other aspects of the child that only a parent can know. They can listen to what the other team members think their child needs to work on at school and share their suggestions. They can also report on whether the skills the child is learning at school are being used at home. (See the information at the end of this section about parents' possible need for an interpreter.)

Teachers are vital participants in the IEP meeting as well. At least one of the child's *regular education teachers* must be on the IEP team if the child is (or may be) participating in the regular education environment. The regular education teacher has a great deal to share with the team. For example, he or she might talk about:

- the general curriculum in the regular classroom;

155

- the aids, services, or changes to the educational program that would help the child learn and achieve; and
- strategies to help the child with behavior, if behavior is an issue.
- The regular education teacher may also discuss with the IEP team the supports for school staff that are needed so that the child can:

  - advance toward his or her annual goals;
  - be involved and progress in the general curriculum;
  - participate in extracurricular and other activities; and
  - be educated with other children, both with and without disabilities.

Supports for school staff may include professional development or more training. Professional development and training are important for teachers, administrators, bus drivers, cafeteria workers, and others who provide services for children with disabilities.

Extra Information: The Regular Education Teacher as Part of the IEP Team

Appendix A of the federal regulations for Part B of IDEA answers many questions about the IEP. Question 24 addresses the role of the regular education teacher on the IEP team. Here's an excerpt from the answer:

"...while a regular education teacher must be a member of the IEP team if the child is, or may be, participating in the regular education environment, the teacher need not (depending upon the child's needs and the purpose of the specific IEP team meeting) be required to participate in all decisions made as part of the meeting or to be present throughout the entire meeting or attend every meeting. For example, the regular education teacher who is a member of the IEP team must participate in discussions and decisions about how to modify the general curriculum in the regular classroom to ensure the child's involvement and progress in the general curriculum and participation in the regular education environment.

"Depending upon the specific circumstances, however, it may not be necessary for the regular education teacher to participate in discussions and decisions regarding, for example, the physical therapy needs of the child, if the teacher is not responsible for implementing that portion of the child's IEP.

"In determining the extent of the regular education teacher's participation at IEP meetings, public agencies and parents should discuss and try to reach agreement on whether the child's regular education teacher that is a member of the IEP team should be present at a particular IEP meeting and, if so, for what period of time. The extent to which it would be appropriate for the regular education teacher member of the IEP team to participate in IEP meetings must be decided on a case-by-case basis."

****

The child's *special education teacher* contributes important information and experience about how to educate children with disabilities. Because of his or her training in special education, this teacher can talk about such issues as:

■ how to modify the general curriculum to help the child learn;
■ the supplementary aids and services that the child may need to be successful in the regular classroom and elsewhere;
■ how to modify testing so that the student can show what he or she has learned; and
■ other aspects of individualizing instruction to meet the student's unique needs.

157

- Beyond helping to write the IEP, the special educator has responsibility for working with the student to carry out the IEP. He or she may:

  - work with the student in a resource room or special class devoted to students receiving special education services;
  - team teach with the regular education teacher; and
  - work with other school staff, particularly the regular education teacher, to provide expertise about addressing the child's unique needs.

Another important member of the IEP team is the *individual who can interpret what the child's evaluation results mean* in terms of designing appropriate instruction. The evaluation results are very useful in determining how the child is currently doing in school and what areas of need the child has. This IEP team member must be able to talk about the instructional implications of the child's evaluation results, which will help the team plan appropriate instruction to address the child's needs.

The *individual representing the school system* is also a valuable team member. This person knows a great deal about special education services and educating children with disabilities. He or she can talk about the necessary school resources. It is important that this individual have the authority to commit resources and be able to ensure that whatever services are set out in the IEP will actually be provided.

The IEP team may also include additional *individuals with knowledge or special expertise about the child*. The parent or the school system can invite these individuals to participate on the team. Parents, for example, may invite an advocate who knows the child, a professional with special expertise about the child and his or her disability, or others (such as a vocational educator who has been working with the child) who can talk about the child's strengths and/or needs. The school system may invite one or more individuals who can offer special expertise or knowledge about the child, such as a paraprofessional or related services professional. Because an important part of developing an IEP is considering a child's need for related services (see the list of related services at the end of this section), related service professionals are often involved as IEP team members or participants. They share their special expertise about the child's needs and how their own professional services can address those needs. Depending on the child's individual needs, some related service professionals attending the IEP meeting or otherwise helping to develop the IEP might include occupational or physical therapists, adaptive physical education providers, psychologists, or speech-language pathologists.

When an IEP is being developed for a student of transition age, *representatives from transition service agencies* can be important participants. (For more information about transition, see the information provided at the end of this section.) Whenever a purpose of meeting is to consider needed transition services, the school must invite a representative of any other agency that is likely to be responsible for providing or paying for transition services. This individual can help the team plan any transition services the student needs. He or she can also commit the resources of the agency to pay for or provide needed transition services. If he or she does not attend the meeting, then the school must take alternative steps to obtain the agency's participation in the planning of the student's transition services.

And, last but not least, the *student* may also be a member of the IEP team. If transition service needs or transition services are going to be discussed at the meeting, the student *must* be invited to attend. More and more students are participating in and even leading their own IEP meetings. This allows them to have a strong voice in their own education and can teach them a great deal about self-advocacy and self-determination.

Will Parents Need an Interpreter in Order to Participate Fully?

If the parents have a limited proficiency in English or are deaf, they may need an interpreter in order to understand and be understood. In this case, the school must make reasonable efforts to arrange for an interpreter during meetings pertaining to the child's educational placement. For meetings regarding the development or review of the IEP, the school must take whatever steps are necessary to ensure that parents understand the meetings--including arranging for an interpreter. This provision should help to ensure that parents are not limited in their ability to participate in their child's education because of language or communication barriers.

Therefore, if parents need an interpreter for a meeting to discuss their child's evaluation, eligibility for special education, or IEP, they should let the school know ahead of time. Telling the school in advance allows the school to make arrangements for an interpreter so that parents can participate fully in the meeting.

Transition Services

Transition refers to activities meant to prepare students with disabilities for adult life. This can include developing postsecondary education and career goals, getting work experience while still in school, setting up linkages with adult service providers such as the vocational rehabilitation agency--whatever is appropriate for the student, given his or her interests, preferences, skills, and needs. Statements about the student's transition needs must be included in the IEP after the student reaches a certain age:

- ***Transition planning***, for students beginning at age 14 (and sometimes younger)--involves helping the student plan his or her courses of study (such as advanced placement or vocational education) so that the classes the student takes will lead to his or her post-school goals.
- ***Transition services***, for students beginning at age 16 (and sometimes younger)--involves providing the student with a coordinated set of services to help the student move from school to adult life. Services focus upon the student's needs or interest in such areas as: higher education or training, employment, adult services, independent living, or taking part in the community.

Related Services

A child may require any of the following related services in order to benefit from special education. Related services, as listed under IDEA, include (but are not limited to):

- Audiology services
- Counseling services
- Early identification and assessment of disabilities in children
- Medical services
- Occupational therapy
- Orientation and mobility services
- Parent counseling and training
- Physical therapy
- Psychological services
- Recreation
- Rehabilitation counseling services
- School health services
- Social work services in schools
- Speech-language pathology services
- Transportation

If a child needs a particular related service in order to benefit from special education, the related service professional should be involved in developing the IEP. He or she may be invited by the school or parent to join the IEP team as a person "with knowledge or special expertise about the child."

Writing the IEP

To help decide what special education and related services the student needs, generally the IEP team will begin by looking at the child's evaluation results, such as classroom tests, individual tests given to establish the student's eligibility, and observations by teachers, parents, paraprofessionals, related service providers, administrators, and others. This information will help the team describe the student's "present levels of educational performance" -in other words, how the student is currently doing in school. Knowing how the student is currently performing in school will help the team develop annual goals to address those areas where the student has an identified educational need.

The IEP team must also discuss specific information about the child. This includes:

- the child's strengths;
- the parents' ideas for enhancing their child's education;
- the results of recent evaluations or reevaluations; and
- how the child has done on state and district-wide tests.
- In addition, the IEP team must consider the "special factors" described between the lines below.

- It is important that the discussion of what the child needs be framed around how to help the child:

  - advance toward the annual goals;
  - be involved in and progress in the general curriculum;

162

- participate in extracurricular and nonacademic activities; and
- be educated with and participate with other children with disabilities and nondisabled children.

Special Factors To Consider

Depending on the needs of the child, the IEP team needs to consider what the law calls *special factors*. These include:

- If the child's *behavior* interferes with his or her learning or the learning of others, the IEP team will consider strategies and supports to address the child's behavior.
- If the child has *limited proficiency in English*, the IEP team will consider the child's language needs as these needs relate to his or her IEP.
- If the child is *blind or visually impaired*, the IEP team must provide for instruction in Braille or the use of Braille, unless it determines after an appropriate evaluation that the child does not need this instruction.
- If the child has *communication needs*, the IEP team must consider those needs.
- If the child is *deaf or hard of hearing*, the IEP team will consider his or her language and communication needs. This includes the child's opportunities to communicate directly with classmates and school staff in his or her usual method of communication (for example, sign language).
- The IEP team must always consider the child's need for *assistive technology* devices or services.

For more information about these special factors, see §300.346, presented in Attachment A.

****

Based on the above discussion, the IEP team will then write the child's IEP. This includes the services and supports the school will provide for the child. If the IEP team decides that a child needs a particular device or service (including an intervention, accommodation, or other program modification), the IEP team must write this information in the IEP. As an example, consider a child whose behavior interferes with learning. The IEP team would need to consider positive and effective ways to address that behavior. The team would discuss the positive behavioral interventions, strategies, and supports that the child needs in order to learn how to control or manage his or her behavior. If the team decides that the child needs a particular service (including an intervention, accommodation, or other program modification), they must include a statement to that effect in the child's IEP.

Deciding Placement

In addition, the child's *placement* (where the IEP will be carried out) must be decided. The placement decision is made by a group of people, including the parents and others who know about the child, what the evaluation results mean, and what types of placements are appropriate. In some states, the IEP team serves as the group making the placement decision. In other states, this decision may be made by another group of people. *In all cases, the parents have the right to be members of the group that decides the educational placement of the child.*

Placement decisions must be made according to IDEA's least restrictive environment requirements--commonly known as LRE. These requirements state that, to the maximum extent appropriate, children with disabilities must be educated with children who do not have disabilities.

The law also clearly states that special classes, separate schools, or other removal of children with disabilities from the regular educational environment may occur only if the nature or severity of the child's disability is such that

164

education in regular classes with the use of supplementary aids and services cannot be achieved satisfactorily.

What type of placements are there? Depending on the needs of the child, his or her IEP may be carried out in the regular class (with supplementary aids and services, as needed), in a special class (where every student in the class is receiving special education services for some or all of the day), in a special school, at home, in a hospital and institution, or in another setting. A school system may meet its obligation to ensure that the child has an appropriate placement available by:

- providing an appropriate program for the child on its own;
- contracting with another agency to provide an appropriate program; or
- utilizing some other mechanism or arrangement that is consistent with IDEA for providing or paying for an appropriate program for the child.

The placement group will base its decision on the IEP and which placement option is appropriate for the child. Can the child be educated in the regular classroom, with proper aids and supports? If the child cannot be educated in the regular classroom, even with appropriate aids and supports, then the placement group will talk about other placements for the child.

After the IEP is Written

When the IEP has been written, parents must receive a copy at no cost to themselves. The IDEA also stresses that everyone who will be involved in *implementing* the IEP must have access to the document. This includes the child's:

- regular education teacher(s);

- special education teacher(s);
- related service provider(s) (for example, speech therapist); or
- any other service provider (such as a paraprofessional) who will be responsible for a part of the child's education.

Each of these individuals needs to know what his or her specific responsibilities are for carrying out the child's IEP. This includes the specific accommodations, modifications, and supports that the child must receive, according to the IEP.

Parents' Permission

Before the school can provide a child with special education and related services *for the first time*, the child's parents must give their written permission.

Implementing the IEP

Once the IEP is written, it is time to carry it out--in other words, to provide the student with the special education and related services as listed in the IEP. This includes all supplementary aids and services and program modifications that the IEP team has identified as necessary for the student to advance appropriately toward his or her IEP goals, to be involved in and progress in the general curriculum, and participate in other school activities. While it is beyond the scope of this guide to discuss in detail the many issues involved in implementing a student's IEP, certain suggestions can be offered.

- Every individual involved in providing services to the student should know and understand his or her responsibilities for carrying out the IEP. This will help ensure that the student receives the services that have been planned, including the specific modifications and accommodations the IEP team has identified as necessary.

- Teamwork plays an important part in carrying out the IEP. Many professionals are likely to be involved in providing services and supports to the student. Sharing expertise and insights can help make everyone's job a lot easier and can certainly improve results for students with disabilities. Schools can encourage teamwork by giving teachers, support staff, and/or paraprofessionals time to plan or work together on such matters as adapting the general curriculum to address the student's unique needs. Teachers, support staff, and others providing services for children with disabilities may request training and staff development.

- Communication between home and school is also important. Parents can share information about what is happening at home and build upon what the child is learning at school. If the child is having difficulty at school, parents may be able to offer insight or help the school explore possible reasons as well as possible solutions.

- It is helpful to have someone in charge of coordinating and monitoring the services the student receives. In addition to special education, the student may be receiving any number of related services. Many people may be involved in delivering those services. Having a person in charge of overseeing that services are being delivered as planned can help ensure that the IEP is being carried out appropriately.

- The regular progress reports that the law requires will help parents and schools monitor the child's progress toward his or her annual goals. It is important to know if the child is not making the progress expected-or if he or she has progressed much faster than expected. Together, parents and school personnel can then address the child's needs as those needs become evident.

167

Reviewing and Revising the IEP

The IEP team must review the child's IEP at least once a year. One purpose of this review is to see whether the child is achieving his or her annual goals. The team must revise the child's individualized education program, if necessary, to address:

- the child's progress or lack of expected progress toward the annual goals and in the general curriculum;
- information gathered through any reevaluation of the child;
- information about the child that the parents share;
- information about the child that the school shares (for example, insights from the teacher based on his or her observation of the child or the child's classwork);
- the child's anticipated needs; or
- other matters.

Although the IDEA requires this IEP review at least once a year, in fact the team may review and revise the IEP more often. Either the parents or the school can ask to hold an IEP meeting to revise the child's IEP. For example, the child may not be making progress toward his or her IEP goals, and his or her teacher or parents may become concerned. On the other hand, the child may have met most or all of the goals in the IEP, and new ones need to be written. In either case, the IEP team would meet to revise the IEP.

Look at Those Factors Again!

When the IEP team is meeting to conduct a review of the child's IEP and, as necessary, to revise it, members must again consider all of the factors discussed under the section "Writing the IEP." This includes:

- the child's strengths,

168

- the parents' ideas for enhancing their child's education,
- the results of recent evaluations or reevaluations, and
- how the child has done on state and district-wide tests.

The IEP team must also consider the "special factors," as listed in that section.

What If Parents Don't Agree With the IEP?

There are times when parents may not agree with the school's recommendations about their child's education. Under the law, parents have the right to challenge decisions about their child's eligibility, evaluation, placement, and the services that the school provides to the child. If parents disagree with the school's actions--or refusal to take action--in these matters, they have the right to pursue a number of options. They may do the following:

- *Try to reach an agreement.* Parents can talk with school officials about their concerns and try to reach an agreement. Sometimes the agreement can be temporary. For example, the parents and school can agree to try a plan of instruction or a placement for a certain period of time and see how the student does.
- *Ask for mediation.* During mediation, the parents and school sit down with someone who is not involved in the disagreement and try to reach an agreement. The school may offer mediation, if it is available as an option for resolving disputes prior to due process.
- *Ask for due process.* During a due process hearing, the parents and school personnel appear before an impartial hearing officer and present their sides of the story. The hearing officer decides how to solve the problem. (Note: Mediation must be available at least at the time a due process hearing is requested.)
- *File a complaint with the state education agency.* To file a complaint, generally parents write directly to the SEA and say what part of IDEA they believe the school

169

has violated. The agency must resolve the complaint within 60 calendar days. An extension of that time limit is permitted only if exceptional circumstances exist with respect to the complaint.

OSEP Monitoring

The U.S. Department of Education's Office of Special Education Programs (OSEP) regularly monitors states to see that they are complying with IDEA. Every two years OSEP requires that states report progress toward meeting established performance goals that, at a minimum, address the performance of children on assessments, drop--out rates, and graduation rates. As part of its monitoring, the Department reviews IEPs *and* interviews parents, students, and school staff to find out:

- whether, and how, the IEP team made the decisions reflected in the IEP;
- whether those decisions and the IEP content are based on the child's unique needs, as determined through evaluation and the IEP process;
- whether any state or local policies or practices have interfered with decisions of the IEP team about the child's educational needs and the services that the school would provide to meet those needs; and
- whether the school has provided the services listed in the IEP.

This guide is intended to help states and school districts write IEPs that comply with IDEA. Writing effective IEPs is a very important first step in improving educational results for children with disabilities.

Summary

The IEP is the cornerstone of special education. Writing and implementing an effective IEP involves many people, many different steps, and collaborative decision making.

The information provided in this guide about the IEP has been fairly general. To help you get better acquainted with the various parts of the IEP, a sample IEP form is presented on the next pages. The sample IEP form includes space for all of the information that an IEP must contain under federal law. (Remember that IEP forms in your area may require more information that may be of value to the student and those implementing the IEP.) The different parts of the sample are paired with direct quotes from the law, so that you can easily see:

- how the law defines what type of information goes into the various parts of a child's IEP, and
- how this information goes together to create an educational program for a particular child.

Attachment A presents the IDEA's regulations for "Individualized Education Programs" (§§300.340-300.350). Under §300.347, where "IEP content" is described, we have included additional information primarily from Appendix A and Attachment 1 of the regulations. This information can be very useful in developing a fuller understanding of what type of information is important to capture about a child in the IEP.

Use of this IEP form, or any other form, will not, in and of itself, ensure compliance with IDEA's Part B requirements. Whether or not a state or local education agency chooses to require or recommend that teams use this form for IEPs, all IEP team participants including parents need to receive clear guidance and training regarding Part B requirements and to understand the importance of the IEP in focusing instruction to meet the unique needs of each child with a disability.

[Page 1 of 5]

Sample Form

Individualized Education Program (IEP)

Student Name   [Space to write]

Date of Meeting to Develop or Review IEP

[Space to write]

Note: For each student with a disability beginning at age 14 (or younger, if appropriate), a statement of the student's transition service needs must be included under the applicable parts of the IEP. The statement must focus on the courses the student needs to take to reach his or her post-school goals.

****

From the Regulations:

Statement of Transition Service Needs--34 CFR §300.347(b)(1)

"The IEP must include...[f]or each student with a disability beginning at age 14 (or younger, if determined appropriate by the IEP team), and updated annually, a statement of the transition service needs of the student under the applicable components of the student's IEP that focuses on the student's courses of study (such as participation in advanced- placement courses or a vocational education program);"

****

Present Levels of Educational Performance

[Space to write]

****

From the Regulations:

Statement of Present Levels of Educational Performance--34 CFR §300.347(a)(1)

"The IEP for each child with a disability must include . . . a statement of the child's present levels of educational performance, including

> "(i) How the child's disability affects the child's involvement and progress in the general curriculum (i.e., the same curriculum as for nondisabled children), or

> "(ii) For preschool children, as appropriate, how the disability affects the child's participation in appropriate activities;"

****

[Page 2 of 5]

Measurable Annual Goals (Including Benchmarks or Short-Term Objectives)

[space to write]

From the Regulations:

Statement of Measurable Annual Goals, Including Benchmarks or Short-Term

Objectives--34 CFR §300.347(a)(2)

"The IEP for each child with a disability must include . . . a statement of measurable annual goals, including benchmarks or short-term objectives, related to

"(i)   Meeting the child's needs that result from the child's disability to enable the child to be involved in and progress in the general curriculum (i.e., the same curriculum as for nondisabled children), or for preschool children, as appropriate, to participate in appropriate activities; and

"(ii)   Meeting each of the child's other educational needs that result from the child's disability;"

****

Special Education and Related Services

[space to write]

- Start Date   [space to write]
- Location   [space to write]
- Frequency   [space to write]
- Duration   [space to write]

Supplementary Aids and Services

[space to write]

- Start Date   [space to write]
- Location   [space to write]
- Frequency   [space to write]
- Duration   [space to write]

Program Modifications or Supports for School Personnel
[space to write]

- Start Date   [space to write]
- Location   [space to write]
- Frequency   [space to write]
- Duration   [space to write]

****

From the Regulations:

Statement of the Special Education and Related Services, Supplementary Aids and Services, Program Modifications, and Supports For School Personnel--34 CFR §300.347(a)(3)

"The IEP for each child with a disability must include... a statement of the special education and related services and supplementary aids and services to be provided to the child, or on behalf of the child, and a statement of the program modifications or supports for school personnel that will be provided for the child

"(i) To advance appropriately toward attaining the annual goals;

"(ii) To be involved and progress in the general curriculum in accordance with 34 CFR §300.347(a)(1) and to participate in extracurricular and other nonacademic activities; and

"(iii)To be educated and participate with other children with disabilities and nondisabled children in the activities described in this section;"

--ALSO--

Beginning Date, Frequency, Location, and Duration of Services and Modifications--

34 CFR §300.347(a)(6)

"The IEP for each child with a disability must include . . . the projected date for the beginning of the services and modifications described in 34 CFR §300.347(a)(3), and the anticipated frequency, location, and duration of those services and modifications;"

****

[Page 3 of 5]

Explanation of Extent, if Any, to Which Child Will Not Participate with Nondisabled Children

[space to write]

****

From the Regulations:

Explanation of Extent, if Any, to Which Child Will Not Participate with Nondisabled Children

34 CFR §300.347(a)(4)

"The IEP for each child with a disability must include . . . an explanation of the extent, if any, to which the child will not participate with nondisabled children in the regular class and in the activities described in 34 CFR §300.347(a)(3);"

****

Administration of State and District-wide Assessments of Student Achievement

Any Individual Modifications In Administration Needed For Child To Participate In State Or District-wide Assessment(s)

[space to write]

****

From the Regulations:

Statement Of Any Individual Modifications in Administration of State or District-wide Assessments 34--CFR §300.347(a)(5)(i)

"The IEP for each child with a disability must include . . . a statement of any individual modifications in the administration of State or district-wide assessments of student achievement that are needed in order for the child to participate in the assessment;"

****

If IEP Team Determines That Child Will Not Participate In A Particular State Or District-Wide Assessment

■ Why isn't the assessment appropriate for the child?
[space to write]
■ How will the child be assessed?
[space to write]

****

From the Regulations:

177

If Child Will Not Participate in State or District-wide Assessment--34 CFR §300.347(a)(5)(ii)

"If the IEP team determines that a child with a disability will not participate in a particular State or district-wide assessment of student achievement (or part of an assessment), the IEP must include a statement of

"(A) Why that assessment is not appropriate for the child; and

"(B) How the child will be assessed;"

[Page 4 of 5]

How Child's Progress Toward Annual Goals Will Be Measured

[space to write]

****

From the Regulations:

How Child's Progress Will Be Measured--34 CFR §300.347(a)(7)(i)

"The IEP for each child with a disability must include . . . a statement of how the child's progress toward the annual goals described in 34 CFR §300.347(a)(2) will be measured;"

****

How Child's Parents Will Be Regularly Informed Of Child's Progress Toward Annual Goals And Extent To Which Child's Progress Is Sufficient To Meet Goals By End of Year

[space to write]

****

From the Regulations:

How Parents Will Be Informed of Their Child's Progress--34 CFR §300.347(a)(7)(ii)

"The IEP for each child with a disability must include . . . a statement of how the child's parents will be regularly informed (through such means as periodic report cards), at least as often as parents are informed of their nondisabled children's progress, of

"(A) Their child's progress toward the annual goals; and

"(B) The extent to which that progress is sufficient to enable the child to achieve the goals by the end of the year."

****

[Page 5 of 5]

(Beginning at age 16 or younger if determined appropriate by IEP team)

Statement of Needed Transition Services, Including, If Appropriate, Statement Of Interagency Responsibilities Or Any Needed Linkages

[space to write]

****

From the Regulations:

Statement of Needed Transition Services--34 CFR §300.347(b)(2)

"The IEP must include . . . for each student with a disability beginning at age 16 (or younger, if determined appropriate by the IEP team), a statement of needed transition services for the student, including, if appropriate, a statement of the interagency responsibilities or any needed linkages."

Definition of "Transition Services"--34 CFR §300.29

"(a) As used in [Part B], "transition services" means a coordinated set of activities for a student with a disability that:

"(1) Is designed within an outcome-oriented process, that promotes movement from school to post-school activities, including post-secondary education, vocational training, integrated employment (including supported employment), continuing and adult education, adult services, independent living, or community participation;

"(2) Is based on the individual student's needs, taking into account the student's preferences and interests; and

"(3) Includes: (i) Instruction; (ii) Related services; (iii) Community experiences; (iv) The development of employment and other post-school adult living objectives; and (v) If appropriate, acquisition of daily living skills and functional vocational evaluation.

"(b) Transition services for students with disabilities may be special education, if provided as specially designed instruction or related services, if required to assist a student with a disability to benefit from special education."

****

(In a state that transfers rights to the student at the age of majority, the following information must be included

180

beginning at least one year before the student reaches the age of majority)

The student has been informed of the rights under Part B of IDEA, if any, that will transfer to the student on reaching the age of majority.   Yes [box to check]

****

From the Regulations:

Age of Majority--34 CFR §300.347(c)

"In a State that transfers rights at the age majority, beginning at least one year before a student reaches the age of majority under State law, the student's IEP must include a statement that the student has been informed of his or her rights under Part B of the Act, if any, that will transfer to the student on reaching the age of majority, consistent with 34 CFR §300.517."

****

Information Resources

If you would like more information about special education, children with disabilities, the IEP process, or the IDEA, contact your state education agency or your local education agency. Additional sources of information include the following:

Office of Special Education Programs
Office of Special Education and Rehabilitative Services
U.S. Department of Education
Mary E. Switzer Building
330 C Street SW
Washington, DC 20202
(202) 205-5507 (Voice/TTY)
Web: www.ed.gov/offices/OSERS/OSEP

National Information Center for Children and Youth with Disabilities (NICHCY)
P.O. Box 1492
Washington, DC 20013
(800) 695-0285 (Voice/TTY); (202) 884-8200 (V/TTY)
E-mail: nichcy@aed.org
Web: www.nichcy.org

ERIC Clearinghouse on Disabilities and Gifted Education (ERIC EC)
1920 Association Drive
Reston, VA 20191-1589
(800) 328-0272
E-mail: ericec@cec.sped.org
Web: http://ericec.org

Technical Assistance for Parent Centers--the Alliance
PACER Center
4826 Chicago Avenue South
Minneapolis, MN 55417-1098
(888) 248-0822; (612) 827-2966
(612) 827-7770 (TTY)
E-mail: alliance@taalliance.org
Web: www.taalliance.org

The IDEA Partnership Projects

Associations of Service Providers Implementing IDEA Reforms in Education (ASPIIRE)
The Council for Exceptional Children
1920 Association Drive
Reston, VA 20191-1589
(888) 232-7733; (703) 264-9456
(703) 264-9446 (TTY)
E-mail: ideapractices@cec.sped.org
Web: www.ideapractices.org

Families and Advocates Partnerships for Education (FAPE)
PACER Center
4826 Chicago Avenue South
Minneapolis, MN 55417-1098
(888) 248-0822; (612) 827-2966; (612) 827-7770 (TTY)
E-mail: fape@pacer.org
Web: www.fape.org

IDEA Local Implementations by Local Administrators (ILIAD)
The Council for Exceptional Children
1920 Association Drive
Reston, VA 20191-1589
(877) CEC-IDEA; (703) 264-9418; (703) 264-9480 (TTY)
E-mail: ideapractices@cec.sped.org
Web: www.ideapractices.org

The Policy Maker Partnership (PMP) for Implementing IDEA 97
National Association of State Directors of Special
Education
1800 Diagonal Road, Suite 320
Alexandria, VA 22314
(703) 519-3800; (703) 519-7008 (TTY)
E-mail: nasdse@nasdse.org
Web: www.nasdse.org

Regional Resource Centers

Northeast Regional Resource Center (NERRC)
Learning Innovations
20 Winter Sport Lane
Williston, VT 05495
(802) 951-8226; (802) 951-8213 (TTY)
E-mail: nerrc@aol.com
Web: http://www.trinityvt.edu/nerrc
Serving: Connecticut, Maine, Massachusetts, New
Hampshire, New Jersey, New York, Rhode Island, and
Vermont.

Mid-South Regional Resource Center (MSRRC)
Human Development Institute
University of Kentucky
126 Mineral Industries Building
Lexington, KY 40506-0051
(859) 257-4921; (859) 257-2903 (TTY)
E-mail: msrrc@ihdi.uky.edu
Web: http://www.ihdi.uky.edu/msrrc
Serving: Delaware, Kentucky, Maryland, North Carolina,
South Carolina, Tennessee, Virginia, Washington, DC, and
West Virginia.

Southeast Regional Resource Center (SERRC)
School of Education
Auburn University Montgomery
P.O. Box 244023
Montgomery, AL 36124
(334) 244-3100; (334) 244-3800 (TTY)
E-mail: bbeale@edla.aum.edu
Web: http://edla.aum.edu/serrc/serrc.html
Serving: Alabama, Arkansas, Florida, Georgia, Louisiana, Mississippi, Oklahoma, Puerto Rico, Texas, and the U.S. Virgin Islands.

Great Lakes Area Regional Resource Center (GLARRC)
OSU Center for Special Needs
700 Ackerman Road, Suite 440
Columbus, OH 43202
(614) 447-0844; (614) 447-8776 (TTY)
E-mail: daniels.121@osu.edu
Web: http://www.csnp.ohio-state.edu/glarrc.htm
Serving: Illinois, Indiana, Iowa, Michigan, Minnesota, Missouri, Ohio, Pennsylvania, and Wisconsin.

Mountain Plains Regional Resource Center (MPRRC)
Utah State University
1780 North Research Parkway, Suite 112
Logan, UT 84341
(435) 752-0238; (435) 753-9750 (TTY)
E-mail: cope@cc.usu.edu
Web: http://www.usu.edu/mprrc
Serving: Arizona, Bureau of Indian Affairs, Colorado, Kansas, Montana, Nebraska, New Mexico, North Dakota, South Dakota, Utah, and Wyoming.

Western Regional Resource Center (WRRC)
1268 University of Oregon
Eugene, OR 97403-1268
(541) 346-5641; (541) 346-0367 (TTY)
E-mail: wrrc@oregon.uoregon.edu
Web: http://interact.uoregon.edu/wrrc/wrrc.html
Serving: Alaska, American Samoa, California,
Commonwealth of the Northern Mariana Islands, Federated
states of Micronesia, Guam, Hawaii, Idaho, Nevada,
Oregon, Republic of the Marshall Islands, Republic of
Palau, and Washington.

Attachment A

Final Regulations for IEPs:
§§ 300.340--300.350

Attachment A presents the Federal regulations for Individualized Education Programs (IEP). These regulations cover areas such as IEP meetings; the IEP team; parent participation; and the development, review, and revision of the IEP.

Under §300.347--"Content of IEP"--we have included additional guidance on the various parts of the IEP. Generally, this guidance comes from Appendix A and Attachment 1 of the federal regulations for IDEA, which were published March 12, 1999, in the *Federal Register*.

This extra information is intended to highlight and clarify what information needs to be included in a child's IEP.

Individualized Education Programs

§ 300.340 Definitions related to IEPs.

(a) *Individualized education program.* As used in this part, the term *individualized education program or IEP* means a written statement for a child with a disability that is developed, reviewed, and revised in a meeting in accordance with §§ 300.341-300.350.

(b) *Participating agency.* As used in § 300.348, *participating agency* means a State or local agency, other than the public agency responsible for a student's education, that is financially and legally responsible for providing transition services to the student.

(Authority: 20 U.S.C. 1401(11), 1312(a)(10)(B))

§ 300.341 Responsibility of SEA and other public agencies for IEPs.

(a) The SEA shall ensure that each public agency--

(1) Except as provided in §§ 300.450-300.462, develops and implements an IEP for each child with a disability served by that agency; and

(2) Ensures that an IEP is developed and implemented for each eligible child placed in or referred to a private school or facility by the public agency.

(b) Paragraph (a) of this section applies to--

(1) The SEA, if it is involved in providing direct services to children with disabilities, in accordance with

300.370(a) and (b)(1); and

(2) Except as provided in § 300.600(d), the other public agencies described in § 300.2, including LEAs and other State agencies that provide special education and related services either directly, by contract, or through other arrangements.

(Authority: 20 U.S.C. 1412(a)(4), (a)(10)(B))

§ 300.342 When IEPs must be in effect.

(a) *General.* At the beginning of each school year, each public agency shall have an IEP in effect for each child with a disability within its jurisdiction.

(b) *Implementation of IEPs.* Each public agency shall ensure that--

(1) An IEP--

(i) Is in effect before special education and related services are provided to an eligible child under this part; and

(ii) Is implemented as soon as possible following the meetings described under § 300.343;

(2) The child's IEP is accessible to each regular education teacher, special education teacher, related service provider, and other service provider who is responsible for its implementation; and

(3) Each teacher and provider described in paragraph (b)(2) of this section is informed of--

(i) His or her specific responsibilities related to implementing the child's IEP; and

(ii) The specific accommodations, modifications, and supports that must be provided for the child in accordance with the IEP.

(c) *IEP or IFSP for children aged 3 through 5.*

(1) In the case of a child with a disability aged 3 through 5 (or, at the discretion of the SEA a 2-year-old child with a disability who will turn age 3 during the school year), an IFSP that contains the material described in section 636 of the Act, and that is developed in accordance with 300.341- 300.346 and 300.349-300.350, may serve as the IEP of the child if using that plan as the IEP is--

(i) Consistent with State policy; and

(ii) Agreed to by the agency and the child's parents.

(2) In implementing the requirements of paragraph (c)(1) of this section, the public agency shall--

(i) Provide to the child's parents a detailed explanation of the differences between an IFSP and an IEP; and

(ii) If the parents choose an IFSP, obtain written informed consent from the parents.

(d) *Effective date for new requirements.* All IEPs developed, reviewed, or revised on or after July 1, 1998 must meet the requirements of §§ 300.340- 300.350.

(Authority: 20 U.S.C. 1414(d)(2)(A) and (B), Pub. L. 105-17, sec. 201(a)(2)(A), (C)

§ 300.343 IEP meetings.

(a) *General.* Each public agency is responsible for initiating and conducting meetings for the purpose of developing, reviewing, and revising the IEP of a child with a disability (or, if consistent with § 300.342(c), an IFSP).

(b) *Initial IEPs; provision of services.* (1) Each public agency shall ensure that within a reasonable period of time following the agency's receipt of parent consent to an initial evaluation of a child--

(i) The child is evaluated; and

(ii) If determined eligible under this part, special education and related services are made available to the child in accordance with an IEP.

(2) In meeting the requirement in paragraph (b)(1) of this section, a meeting to develop an IEP for the child must be conducted within 30 days of a determination that the child needs special education and related services.

(c) *Review and revision of IEPs.* Each public agency shall ensure that the IEP team-

(1) Reviews the child's IEP periodically, but not less than annually, to determine whether the annual goals for the child are being achieved; and

(2) Revises the IEP as appropriate to address--

(i) Any lack of expected progress toward the annual goals described in § 300.347(a), and in the general curriculum, if appropriate;

(ii) The results of any reevaluation conducted under § 300.536;

(iii) Information about the child provided to, or by, the parents, as described in 300.533(a)(1);

(iv) The child's anticipated needs; or

(v) Other matters.

(Authority: 20 U.S.C. 1413(a)(1), 1414(d)(4)(A))

§ 300.344 IEP team.

(a) *General.* The public agency shall ensure that the IEP team for each child with a disability includes-

(1) The parents of the child;

(2) At least one regular education teacher of the child (if the child is, or may be, participating in the regular education environment);

(3) At least one special education teacher of the child, or if appropriate, at least one special education provider of the child;

(4) A representative of the public agency who--

(i) Is qualified to provide, or supervise the provision of, specially designed instruction to meet the unique needs of children with disabilities;

(ii) Is knowledgeable about the general curriculum; and

(iii) Is knowledgeable about the availability of resources of the public agency;

(5) An individual who can interpret the instructional implications of evaluation results, who may be a member of the team described in paragraphs (a)(2) through (6) of this section;

(6) At the discretion of the parent or the agency, other individuals who have knowledge or special expertise

regarding the child, including related services personnel as appropriate; and

(7) If appropriate, the child.

(b) *Transition services participants.* (1) Under paragraph (a)(7) of this section, the public agency shall invite a student with a disability of any age to attend his or her IEP meeting if a purpose of the meeting will be the consideration of-

(i) The student's transition services needs under § 300.347(b)(1);

(ii) The needed transition services for the student under § 300.347(b)(2); or

(iii) Both.

(2) If the student does not attend the IEP meeting, the public agency shall take other steps to ensure that the student's preferences and interests are considered.

(3)(i) In implementing the requirements of 300.347(b)(2), the public agency also shall invite a representative of any other agency that is likely to be responsible for providing or paying for transition services.

(ii) If an agency invited to send a representative to a meeting does not do so, the public agency shall take other steps to obtain participation of the other agency in the planning of any transition services.

(c) *Determination of knowledge and special expertise.* The determination of the knowledge or special expertise of any individual described in paragraph (a)(6) of this section shall be made by the party (parents or public agency) who invited the individual to be a member of the IEP.

(d) *Designating a public agency representative.* A public agency may designate another public agency member of the IEP team to also serve as the agency representative, if the criteria in paragraph (a)(4) of this section are satisfied.

(Authority: 20 U.S.C. 1401(30), 1414(d)(1)(A)(7), (B))

§ 300.345 Parent participation.

(a) *Public agency responsibility-general.* Each public agency shall take steps to ensure that one or both of the parents of a child with a disability are present at each IEP meeting or are afforded the opportunity to participate, including--

(1) Notifying parents of the meeting early enough to ensure that they will have an opportunity to attend; and

(2) Scheduling the meeting at a mutually agreed on time and place.

(b) *Information provided to parents.* (1) The notice required under paragraph (a)(1) of this section must-

(i) Indicate the purpose, time, and location of the meeting and who will be in attendance; and

(ii) Inform the parents of the provisions in 300.344(a)(6) and (c) (relating to the participation of other individuals on the IEP team who have knowledge or special expertise about the child).

(2) For a student with a disability beginning at age 14, or younger, if appropriate, the notice must also--

(i) Indicate that a purpose of the meeting will be the development of a statement of the transition services needs of the student required in

194

300.347(b)(1); and

(ii) Indicate that the agency will invite the student.

(3) For a student with a disability beginning at age 16, or younger, if appropriate, the notice must--

(i) Indicate that a purpose of the meeting is the consideration of needed transition services for the student required in § 300.347(b)(2);

(ii) Indicate that the agency will invite the student; and

(iii) Identify any other agency that will be invited to send a representative.

(c) *Other methods to ensure parent participation.* If neither parent can attend, the public agency shall use other methods to ensure parent participation, including individual or conference telephone calls.

(d) *Conducting an IEP meeting without a parent in attendance.* A meeting may be conducted without a parent in attendance if the public agency is unable to convince the parents that they should attend. In this case the public agency must have a record of its attempts to arrange a mutually agreed on time and place, such as--

(1) Detailed records of telephone calls made or attempted and the results of those calls;

(2) Copies of correspondence sent to the parents and any responses received; and

(3) Detailed records of visits made to the parent's home or place of employment and the results of those visits.

(e) *Use of interpreters or other action, as appropriate.* The public agency shall take whatever action is necessary to ensure that the parent understands the proceedings at the

IEP meeting, including arranging for an interpreter for parents with deafness or whose native language is other than English.

(f) *Parent copy of child's IEP*. The public agency shall give the parent a copy of the child's IEP at no cost to the parent.

(Authority: 20 U.S.C. 1414(d)(1)(B)(i))

§ 300.346 Development, review, and revision of IEP.

(a) *Development of IEP. (1) General*. In developing each child's IEP, the IEP team, shall consider-

(i) The strengths of the child and the concerns of the parents for enhancing the education of their child;

(ii) The results of the initial or most recent evaluation of the child; and

(iii) As appropriate, the results of the child's performance on any general State or district-wide assessment programs.

(2) *Consideration of special factors*. The IEP team also shall-

(i) In the case of a child whose behavior impedes his or her learning or that of others, consider, if appropriate, strategies, including positive behavioral interventions, strategies, and supports to address that behavior;

(ii) In the case of a child with limited English proficiency, consider the language needs of the child as those needs relate to the child's IEP;

(iii) In the case of a child who is blind or visually impaired, provide for instruction in Braille and the use of

Braille unless the IEP team determines, after an evaluation of the child's reading and writing skills, needs, and appropriate reading and writing media (including an evaluation of the child's future needs for instruction in Braille or the use of Braille), that instruction in Braille or the use of Braille is not appropriate for the child;

(iv) Consider the communication needs of the child, and in the case of a child who is deaf or hard of hearing, consider the child's language and communication needs, opportunities for direct communications with peers and professional personnel in the child's language and communication mode, academic level, and full range of needs, including opportunities for direct instruction in the child's language and communication mode; and

(v) Consider whether the child requires assistive technology devices and services.

(b) *Review and Revision of IEP.* In conducting a meeting to review, and, if appropriate, revise a child's IEP, the IEP team shall consider the factors described in paragraph (a) of this section.

(c) *Statement in IEP.* If, in considering the special factors described in paragraphs (a)(1) and (2) of this section, the IEP team determines that a child needs a particular device or service (including an intervention, accommodation, or other program modification) in order for the child to receive FAPE, the IEP team must include a statement to that effect in the child's IEP.

(d) *Requirement with respect to regular education teacher.* The regular education teacher of a child with a disability, as a member of the IEP team, must, to the extent appropriate, participate in the development, review, and revision of the child's IEP, including assisting in the determination of-

(1) Appropriate positive behavioral interventions and strategies for the child; and

(2) Supplementary aids and services, program modifications or supports for school personnel that will be provided for the child, consistent with 300.347(a)(3).

(e) *Construction.* Nothing in this section shall be construed to require the IEP team to include information under one component of a child's IEP that is already contained under another component of the child's IEP.

(Authority: 20 U.S.C. 1414(d)(3) and (4)(B) and (e))

§ 300.347 Content of IEP.

"(a) *General.* The IEP for each child with a disability must include-

"(1) A statement of the child's present levels of educational performance, including-

"(i) How the child's disability affects the child's involvement and progress in the general curriculum (i.e., the same curriculum as for nondisabled children); or

"(ii) For preschool children, as appropriate, how the disability affects the child's participation in appropriate activities;

****

Additional Guidance

An IEP must include measurable annual goals that relate to meeting the child's needs that result from the child's disability to enable the child to be involved in and progress in the general curriculum, and to meeting each of the child's other educational needs that result from the child's disability [34 CFR §300.347(a)(2)]. Thus, if a child's unique needs require goals that address the child's present levels of educational performance in nonacademic areas of instructional need, such as behavioral skills, communication and language skills, self-determination skills, job-related skills, independent living skills, or social skills, the statement of present levels of educational performance in the child's IEP should provide information regarding the child's present levels of educational performance in those areas.

****

"(2) A statement of measurable annual goals, including benchmarks or short-term objectives, related to-

"(i) Meeting the child's needs that result from the child's disability to enable the child to be involved in and progress in the general curriculum (i.e., the same curriculum as for nondisabled children), or for preschool children, as appropriate, to participate in appropriate activities; and

"(ii) Meeting each of the child's other educational needs that result from the child's disability;

****

Additional Guidance

Each annual goal must include either short-term objectives or benchmarks. The purpose of both is to enable a child's teacher(s), parents, and others involved in developing and implementing the child's IEP, to gauge, at intermediate times during the year, how well the child is progressing toward achievement of the annual goal. [Appendix A to 34 CFR Part 300--Notice of Interpretation (Appendix A),

199

Response to Question 1, 64 *Federal Register*, page 12471 (March 12, 1999).]

An IEP team may use either short-term objectives (that generally break the skills described in the annual goal down into discrete components) or benchmarks (which can be thought of as describing the amount of progress the child is expected to make within specified segments of the year), or a combination of the two, depending on the nature of the annual goals and the needs of the child. [Appendix A to 34 CFR Part 300--Notice of Interpretation (Appendix A), Response to Question 1, 64 *Federal Register*, page 12471 (March 12, 1999).]

A child's IEP must include measurable annual goals that relate to meeting the child's needs that result from the child's disability to enable the child to be involved in and progress in the general curriculum, and to meeting each of the child's other educational needs that result from the child's disability [34 CFR §300.347(a)(2)]. This may, depending on the child's needs, include annual goals that relate to the child's needs in such areas as behavioral skills, communication, self-determination skills, job-related skills, independent living skills, or social skills.

A public agency is not required to include in an IEP annual goals that relate to areas of the general curriculum in which the child's disability does not affect the child's ability to be involved in and progress in the general curriculum. If a child needs only modifications or accommodations in order to progress in an area of the general curriculum, the IEP does not need to include a goal for that area; however the IEP would need to specify those modifications or accommodations. [Appendix A, Response to Question 4, 64 *Federal Register*, page 12472 (March 12, 1999).]

****

"(3) A statement of the special education and related services and supplementary aids and services to be provided to the child, or on behalf of the child, and a statement of the program modifications or supports for school personnel that will be provided for the child--

"(i) To advance appropriately toward attaining the annual goals;

"(ii) To be involved and progress in the general curriculum in accordance with paragraph (a)(1) of this section and to participate in extracurricular and other nonacademic activities; and

"(iii) To be educated and participate with other children with disabilities and nondisabled children in the activities described in this section;

Additional Guidance

The type and amount of services to be provided must be stated in the IEP, so that the level of the agency's commitment of resources will be clear to parents and other IEP team members. [Appendix A, Response to Question 35, 64 *Federal Register*, page 12479 (March 12, 1999).]

The amount of time to be committed to each of the various services to be provided must be appropriate to the specific service and stated in the IEP in a manner that is clear to all who are involved in both the development and implementation of the IEP. [Appendix A, Response to Question 35, 64 *Federal Register*, page 12479 (March 12, 1999).]

The amount of a special education or related service to be provided to a child may be stated in the IEP as a range (e.g., speech therapy to be provided three times a week for 30-45 minutes per session) only if the IEP team determines that stating the amount of the services as a range is necessary to meet the unique needs of the child. For

201

example, it would be appropriate for the IEP to specify, based upon the IEP team's determination of the student's unique needs, that particular services are needed only under specific circumstances, such as the occurrence of a seizure or of a particular behavior. A range may not be used because of personnel shortages or uncertainty regarding the availability of staff. [Appendix A, Response to Question 35, 64 *Federal Register*, page 12479 (March 12, 1999).]

The term "on behalf of the child" includes, among other things, services that are provided to the parents or teacher of the child with a disability to help them to more effectively work with the child. . . Supports for school personnel could also include special training for a child's teacher. However, in order for the training to meet the requirements of §300.347(a)(3), it would normally be targeted directly to on assisting the teacher to meet a unique and specific need of the child, and not simply to participate in an inservice training program that is generally available in a public agency. [Attachment 1-Analysis of Comments and Changes (Attachment 1), 64 *Federal Register*, page 12593 (March 12, 1999).]

If the IEP team determines that a child with a disability needs extended school year services to receive a free appropriate public education , the public agency must ensure that the child receives those services. A public agency may not-(i) Limit extended school year services to particular categories of disability; or (ii) Unilaterally limit the type, amount, or duration of those services. 34 CFR §300.309(a).

Section 300.346(a)(1) requires that, in developing each child's IEP, the IEP team, shall consider-(i) The strengths of the child and the concerns of the parents for enhancing the education of their child; (ii) The results of the initial or most recent evaluation of the child; and (iii) As appropriate, the results of the child's performance on any general State or district-wide assessment programs.

Section 300.346(a)(2) requires that the IEP team also:

i. In the case of a child whose behavior impedes his or her learning or that of others, consider, if appropriate, strategies, including positive behavioral interventions, strategies, and supports to address that behavior;

ii. In the case of a child with limited English proficiency, consider the language needs of the child as those needs relate to the child's IEP;

iii. In the case of a child who is blind or visually impaired, provide for instruction in Braille and the use of Braille unless the IEP team determines, after an evaluation of the child's reading and writing skills, needs, and appropriate reading and writing media (including an evaluation of the child's future needs for instruction in Braille or the use of Braille), that instruction in Braille or the use of Braille is not appropriate for the child;

iv. Consider the communication needs of the child, and in the case of a child who is deaf or hard of hearing, consider the child's language and communication needs, opportunities for direct communications with peers and professional personnel in the child's language and communication mode, academic level, and full range of needs, including opportunities for direct instruction in the child's language and communication mode; and

v. Consider whether the child requires assistive technology devices and services.

****

"(4) An explanation of the extent, if any, to which the child will not participate with nondisabled children in the regular class and in the activities described in paragraph (a)(3) of this section;

****

Additional Guidance

The IEP team must consider the extent, if any, to which the child will not participate with nondisabled children in the regular class; the general curriculum; and in extracurricular and other nonacademic activities. If the IEP team determines that the child cannot participate full time with nondisaled children in the regular classroom, the general curriculum, and in extracurricular and other nonacademic activities, the IEP must include a statement that explains why full participation is not possible. [Attachment 1, 64 *Federal Register*, page 12593 (March 12, 1999).]

The IEP team must consider whether or not the child's education can be achieved satisfactorily in the regular classes with the use of supplementary aids and services. The IEP team must consider the full range of supplementary aids and services that if provided, would facilitate the student's placement in the regular classroom. [Appendix A, Response to Question 1, 64 *Federal Register*, page 12471 (March 12, 1999).]

In determining the extent, if any, to which a child with a disability will be removed from the regular educational environment, a public agency must ensure that:

(1) such removal occurs only if the nature or severity of the child's disability is such that education in regular classes with the use of supplementary aids and services cannot be achieved satisfactorily [34 CFR §300.550(b)(2)];

(2) a child with a disability is not removed from education in age-appropriate regular classrooms solely because of needed modifications in the general curriculum [34 CFR §300.552(e)]; and

(3) each child with a disability participates with nondisabled children in nonacademic and extracurricular

services and activities to the maximum extent appropriate (34 CFR §300.553).

****

"(5)(i) A statement of any individual modifications in the administration of State or district-wide assessments of student achievement that are needed in order for the child to participate in the assessment; and

"(ii) If the IEP team determines that the child will not participate in a particular State or district-wide assessment of student achievement (or part of an assessment), a statement of--

"(A) Why that assessment is not appropriate for the child; and

"(B) How the child will be assessed;

Additional Guidance

The IEP for a child with a disability must include a statement of any needed modifications in the administration of State or district-wide assessments, and must, if the IEP team determines that it is not appropriate for the child to participate in a particular assessment, provide a statement of why the particular assessment is not appropriate for the child and how the child will be assessed [34 CFR §300.347(a)(5)]. If the IEP does not indicate any needed modifications or that the particular assessment is not appropriate for the child, this is an indication that the IEP team has determined that the child will participate without modifications in the assessment.

****

"(6) The projected date for the beginning of the services and modifications described in paragraph (a)(3) of this section, and the anticipated frequency, location, and duration of those services and modifications; and

****

Additional Guidance

An IEP that clearly states how often, how long and in what location the public agency will provide the specified services and modifications, and when services and/or modifications will begin meets the requirements of 34 CFR §300.347(a)(6).

****

"(7) A statement of--

"(i) How the child's progress toward the annual goals described in paragraph (a)(2) of this section will be measured; and

"(ii) How the child's parents will be regularly informed (through such means as periodic report cards), at least as often as parents are informed of their nondisabled children's progress, of--

"(A) Their child's progress toward the annual goals; and

"(B) The extent to which that progress is sufficient to enable the child to achieve the goals by the end of the year.

****

Additional Guidance

Each public agency may determine the appropriate method for informing parents of their child's progress. However, the agency "must ensure that whatever methods, or

206

combination of methods, is adopted provides sufficient information to enable parents to be informed of (1) their child's progress toward the annual goals, and (2) the extent to which that progress is sufficient to enable the child to achieve the goals by the end of the year." [Attachment 1, 64 *Federal Register*, page 12594 (March 12, 1999).]

Generally, reports to parents are not expected to be lengthy or burdensome. The statement of the annual goals and short-term objectives or benchmarks in the child's current IEP could serve as the base document for briefly describing the child's progress. [Attachment 1, 64 *Federal Register*, page 12594 (March 12, 1999).]

The IEP team must revise the IEP to address any lack of expected progress toward the annual goals and in the general curriculum [34 CFR §300.343(c)(2)(i)].

****

"(b) *Transition services*. The IEP must include--

"(1) For each student with a disability beginning at age 14 (or younger, if determined appropriate by the IEP team), and updated annually, a statement of the transition service needs of the student under the applicable components of the student's IEP that focuses on the student's courses of study (such as participation in advanced-placement courses or a vocational education program); and

"(2) For each student beginning at age 16 (or younger, if determined appropriate by the IEP team), a statement of needed transition services for the student, including, if appropriate, a statement of the interagency responsibilities or any needed linkages.

****

Additional Guidance

The IEP team, in determining appropriate measurable annual goals (including benchmarks or short term objectives) and services for a student, must determine what instruction and educational experiences will assist the student to prepare for transition for secondary education to post-secondary life. [Appendix A, Response to Question 11, 64 *Federal Register*, page 12474 (March 12, 1999).]

Although the focus of the transition planning process may shift as the student approaches graduation, the IEP team must discuss specific areas beginning at least at age of 14 years, and review these areas annually. [Appendix A, Response to Question 11, 64 *Federal Register*, page 12474 (March 12, 1999).]

If a participating agency, other than the public agency, fails to provide the transition services described in the IEP in accordance with 34 CFR §300.347(b)(1), the public agency shall reconvene the IEP team to identify alternative strategies to meet the transition objective for the student set out in the IEP [34 CFR §300.348(a)].

Nothing in Part B relieves any participating agency, including a State vocational rehabilitation agency, of the responsibility to provide or pay for any transition service that the agency would otherwise provide to students with disabilities who meet the eligibility criteria of that agency [34 CFR §300.348(b)].

If during the course of the IEP meeting, the team identifies additional agencies that are likely to be responsible for providing or paying for transition services for the student, the public agency must determine how it will meet the requirements of §300.344. [Appendix A, Response to Question 13, 64 *Federal Register*, page 12475 (March 12, 1999).]

****

"(c) *Transfer of rights*. In a State that transfers rights at the age majority, beginning at least one year before a student reaches the age of majority under State law, the student's IEP must include a statement that the student has been informed of his or her rights under Part B of the Act, if any, that will transfer to the student on reaching the age of majority, consistent with § 300.517.

****

Additional Guidance

If the public agency receives notice of the student's legal incompetence, so that no rights transfer to the student at the age of majority, the IEP need not include this statement. Attachment 1, 64 *Federal Register*, page 12594 (March 12, 1999).

The IEP could include a description of the rights that have been transferred, but it need not.

****

"(d) *Students with disabilities convicted as adults and incarcerated in adult prisons*. Special rules concerning the content of IEPs for students with disabilities convicted as adults and incarcerated in adult prisons are contained in § 300.311(b) and (c).

(Authority: 20 U.S.C. 1414(d)(1)(A) and (d)(6)(A)(ii))

§ 300.348   Agency responsibilities for transition services.

(a) If a participating agency, other than the public agency, fails to provide the transition services described in the IEP in accordance with § 300.347(b)(1), the public agency shall reconvene the IEP team to identify alternative strategies to meet the transition objectives for the student set out in the IEP.

(b) Nothing in this part relieves any participating agency, including a State vocational rehabilitation agency, of the responsibility to provide or pay for any transition service that the agency would otherwise provide to students with disabilities who meet the eligibility criteria of that agency.

(Authority: 20 U.S.C. 1414(d)(5); 1414(d)(1)(A)(vii))

§ 300.349 Private school placements by public agencies.

(a) *Developing IEPs.* (1) Before a public agency places a child with a disability in, or refers a child to, a private school or facility, the agency shall initiate and conduct a meeting to develop an IEP for the child in accordance with §§ 300.346 and 300.347.

(2) The agency shall ensure that a representative of the private school or facility attends the meeting. If the representative cannot attend, the agency shall use other methods to ensure participation by the private school or facility, including individual or conference telephone calls.

(b) *Reviewing and revising IEPs.* (1) After a child with a disability enters a private school or facility, any meetings to review and revise the child's IEP may be initiated and conducted by the private school or facility at the discretion of the public agency.

(2) If the private school or facility initiates and conducts these meetings, the public agency shall ensure that the parents and an agency representative-

(i) Are involved in any decision about the child's IEP; and

(ii) Agree to any proposed changes in the IEP before those changes are implemented.

(c) *Responsibility*. Even if a private school or facility implements a child's IEP, responsibility for compliance with this part remains with the public agency and the SEA.

(Authority: 20 U.S.C. 1412(a)(10)(B))

§ 300.350 IEP-accountability.

(a) *Provision of services*. Subject to paragraph (b) of this section, each public agency must--

(1) Provide special education and related services to a child with a disability in accordance with the child's IEP; and

(2) Make a good faith effort to assist the child to achieve the goals and objectives or benchmarks listed in the IEP.

(b) *Accountability*. Part B of the Act does not require that any agency, teacher, or other person be held accountable if a child does not achieve the growth projected in the annual goals and benchmarks or objectives. However, the Act does not prohibit a State or public agency from establishing its own accountability systems regarding teacher, school, or agency performance.

(c) *Construction-parent rights*. Nothing in this section limits a parent's right to ask for revisions of the child's IEP or to invoke due process procedures if the parent feels that the efforts required in paragraph (a) of this section are not being made.

(Authority: 20 U.S.C. 1414(d)); Cong. Rec. at H7152 (daily ed., July 21, 1975))